Testimonials

"Your book has been such an inspiration to me. The cool thing is I am still doing what I am supposed to be doing because you made it so easy!"

Cindy S. of Mandeville, LA

"I've read a lot of diet and health books, but this one made sense. It was so easy to understand that I could actually follow the plan."

Lisa T. of Austin, TX

"Short, sweet and to the point! Just the right amount of right information to make achieving my weight loss goal seem easy."

Julie L. of Denver, CO

"A book I could actually read, understand and FINISH! And, a plan I could actually follow. Thank you, Dr. C., for helping me finally get Set on Success!"

Darrell J. of New Orleans, LA

"I've got a lot of weight loss books on my shelf. This one I actually carry with me everyday. It has changed my life."

Joe M. of Phoenix, AZ

"Not only have I lost weight and kept it off, I've done it easily AND with better energy and feeling better than I ever have."

Alice B. of Baton Rouge, LA

"No more diets, no more failures - with this book I am Set on Success and continue on my path of weight loss, wellness and a new sense of vitality."

Kathy M. of Torrington, CT

"Easy to understand, easy to follow... I never believed it could be so simple to finally see the weight loss results I have strived for for so long. Thank you, thank you Dr. Wilbert!"

Sandra H. of Albuquerque, NM

MENDING YOUR METABOLISM

Catherine Wilbert, N.D.

Naturopathic Doctor, Nationally Recognized Wellness Expert

790 Florida Street, Suite 1
Mandeville, LA 70448
888.551.1080
www.catherinewilbert.com

This book is for educational purposes. It is not intended as a substitute for medical advice.
Please consult a qualified health care professional for individual health and medical advice.
The author shall not have any responsibility for any adverse affects arising directly or indirectly
as a result of the information provided in this book.

Throughout this book, trademarked names are used. Rather than put a trademark symbol after
every occurrence of a trademarked name, we use names in an editorial fashion only and to
the benefit of the trademark owner, with no intention of infringement of the trademark. Where
such designations appear in this book, they have been printed with initial capitals.

ISBN 978-0-615-18186-8

MENDING YOUR METABOLISM

Introduction

Congratulations! You've made the commitment to better health. Whether it was the thought of shedding a few pounds to look good, fit better in your clothes, or you are ready to just feel better. Mending Your Metabolism will provide you the tools and just the encouragement you need.

Mending Your Metabolism is a no nonsense, gimmick free approach to end yo-yo dieting and start you on a path to genuine health and wellness. This is much more than just better weight management; it is better energy, better focus, better sleep, and better overall quality of life. Armed with the information in this book you will be able to make better food choices without deprivation, simply by gaining an understanding of what is in what you eat, and what it does in your body. I know many of you are thinking, "Okay, this sounds too simple." The seemingly more obvious solution would be to cut back on the meals and start doing cardio – and lots of it. As much as this may sound unpleasant (at least to most of us), it's bound to burn that extra fat, leaving us lean and toned, ready to show of those abs, right? Wrong! The good news is that these myths about weight loss are just that – while you do need to cut calories and increase activity to lose weight, there is a better, healthier, and more efficient way to do it.

A broken machine cannot be fixed without knowing how it works and so goes mending "a broken metabolism."

First of all, embarking on some crazy fad diet that severely restricts calories may initially produce results, but in the long run will actually slow down your metabolism. Eating more frequent meals throughout the day will actually boost your metabolism. The key is better food choices, balanced meals and portion control.

Unfortunately, the word "diet" has come to have an unpleasant meaning for many people. To some people it means food deprivation and a restricted menu. To others, it stirs up visions of unappetizing and unpalatable food. To almost everyone, diet means a lack of the pleasant, satisfying feeling that comes from a good meal. Diet, however, is very simply what a person eats and drinks every day.

No longer do "healthy" and "tastes great" have to be mutually exclusive. No more deprivation, being hungry, tired and miserable. Gaining an understanding of what is in what you eat is necessary to adopt a "diet" that will not only lead to better weight management, but to a life filled with health and vitality.

Enjoy!

Dr. C's "Set on Success" Tips

First and foremost – this is not a diet, it's not even a drastic lifestyle change. It is an education in a few simple steps to transform your life forever.

1. Baby Steps

This won't be as overwhelming as you may think. An important thing to keep in mind is that you don't have to change your entire lifestyle overnight. Don't put that much pressure on yourself! Making small changes that actually fit into your lifestyle over time will lead to a healthier, happier you. And remember, be consistent. You can't be committed part time. Instead of calling this a diet, call it a gradual lifestyle change. Rather than being focused on strict diets that ultimately only lead to failures, we will focus on one or two small changes that will keep us **Set on Success**!

2. The Food Diary

Let's be honest. When keeping a food diary, write down everything you eat. We all slip up now and then, so if you sneak a chocolate chip cookie, write it down. Had an extra serving of pasta? Write it down. The purpose of your food diary is so you can really see how much you are eating. Writing down what you eat makes you conscious of the foods you are choosing. Be sure to write down the carbs, fats, protein, and calories. This will help you to adjust your meals and show you if you're eating too much of something and not enough of another. At the end of the day add up the numbers. While you don't want to be eating 5000 calories a day, you do want to be more concerned with the quality of the calories than how many you're eating. Calories certainly do count, but not as much as what they are made up of. One hundred calories from eating a cookie is very different from 100

"It's not so much about calories -- as it's what they are made up of."
Dr. C

calories found in a protein shake or grilled chicken breast. Remember to be true to yourself and you will see the results.

3.   Labels, Labels Labels!

Read those labels, and not just the front of the package! Flip it over and examine the nutrition facts panel, and more importantly the ingredients. Remember, the front is the advertising and the back is the truth. While the front may read, "whole grains" or "no trans fats," the back may reveal mostly refined flour or partially hydrogenated ingredients. Know what you're eating. If you can't pronounce most of the ingredients, do you really want to eat them?

4. Portion Control

Buy a food scale and measuring cup. Don't worry, you're not sentenced to be chained to your food scale for life. This will just help you adjust your portions until you know what they should look like. Eventually, you'll be able to use your trained eye to make you truly portion savvy. For those of you who prefer to leave the cooking to your favorite restaurants, this will certainly come in handy. Most restaurants serve up at least double food portions, pile on the carbs, and leave you with very little protein.

5. Out to Eat

When you go out to eat, choose wisely. I know, the half pound burger with fries looks tempting, but so can the mahi mahi with steamed, seasoned veggies! Also, order your food grilled, not deep fried. Get the sauces, dressings and butter on the side. These are where your calories really start to add up. Believe it or not, your food will still taste great when it's not drowning in creams and butter. Just "dipping" will still give you all the flavor, without all the added calories. Ask for your vegetables to be steamed, not sautéed, and hold the butter. Yes, they usually add butter and seasoning to steamed vegetables. Think you're safe with a salad? Not so fast. Most dressings are loaded with bad fats and sugar, even the fat free ones can be loaded with sugar. Be sure to get the dressing on the side and dip your fork into the dressing. Or, ask for olive oil & balsamic vinegar, and use more vinegar than oil. Also, try to stay away from the baskets of bread or chips often served at your table. Usually it is easier to ask your waiter not to bring them, rather than have to overcome the temptation of staring at them, staring at you.

6. Drink your water!

Water! Water, water, water! Water is so very important for almost every function in your body. Try to drink eight pints of water per day. Start with eight, 8 ounce glasses and work your way up. Try adding a slice of lemon or lime for flavor and to increase the ph. You'll be surprised at how easily headaches and fatigue can be stopped with some simple H_2O. And stop drinking away your calories. Research shows that your body does not register liquid and solid calories the same way. If you drink orange juice, your body is still hungry. But if you eat an orange instead, your body will register the calories in a way that makes you begin to feel full. You will also get the benefit of the fiber and other nutrients in the whole fruit. If you want to drink juice, then dilute it with sparkling water. Drink water rather than juice, soda and coffee drinks loaded with milk and/or cream. Research has shown that soft drink consumption is directly correlated to obesity. Diet, *yes diet*, soft drink consumers are at even greater risk! Also, be moderate with liquor. Liquor has absolutely no nutritional value, only empty calories.

7. Don't deprive yourself

Cheating is okay, but in moderation! Allow yourself an "up" day or a cheat meal. You're less likely to call it quits if you allow yourself a little treat every now and then-- not everyday! If you want a juicy hamburger, have one. If you want a slice of pizza, have one. I said a SLICE, not a whole pizza! If you want yogurt, a cookie or a brownie, then go ahead and have one. But don't make a day of it. Just know the calories and predetermine a reasonable portion. That way you won't feel deprived. Also, protein can lower the glycemic index of high carbohydrate foods, so by adding a protein to your "cheat" food, it can lessen its impact. If you do indulge too much one day, don't blow the whole week. Remember, you don't need to wait until Monday to start over. You can start over the next day, or better yet, the next meal!

What's In What You Eat

Introduction

How many diets have you tried? Too many? How many diets required that you eliminate a food group? Some popular diets would have you eliminate, or strongly limit, your carbohydrate intake. Then there are the low or no fat diets that were so popular before the low carb era. Of course, we can't forget the wacky fad diets, like cabbage and cantaloupe, for four excruciating weeks. Well, any diet that requires you to eliminate a food group is not only unhealthy, but will ultimately leave you disappointed. It is not about eliminating a food group, but rather learning how to make better choices within EACH food group. The most important thing to keep in mind when learning how to make better food choices in your lifestyle changes, is that you need all your food groups: proteins, fats, and yes, even carbs. It is also important to understand why these food groups are important and how to choose wisely among them. Menu planning involves more than just counting calories, it involves balancing carbohydrates, proteins and fats. Remember, the quality of your calories count more than the quantity. While calories do count, what those calories are made up of play a much more critical role in successful weight and health management. While it's true that we must expend more energy, or calories, than we take in to lose weight, our bodies are much more complex "chemistry projects" than simple addition and subtraction math equations. Not all calories are equal because of differences in biochemistry and function among carbohydrates, proteins and fats. It is not simply a surplus of calories,

> *"It's not about eliminating a food group – it's making better choices within **each** food group."*

but rather a surplus of calories from certain foods, primarily carbohydrates, that are stored as body fat. If you keep this in mind during your transition a healthier you, you will surely avoid the dreaded yo-yo diet syndrome.

FYI

A "calorie" is defined as the amount of heat (energy) required to raise the temperature of one kilogram of water one-degree centigrade from 15° to 16°C. The values for calories per gram are: 4 calories per gram for carbohydrates, 4 calories per gram for proteins, and 9 calories per gram for fats. Alcohol yields 7 calories per gram.

Protein

Protein - the word itself is a derivative of a Greek word meaning "of primary importance," and whether you are trying to lose weight, gain muscle, or maintain optimum health, the benefits as well as the necessity of protein cannot be overstated. Next to water, protein is the most abundant substance in the human body. All tissues, bones, and nerves are comprised mostly of protein. Your muscles, skin, hair, nails, heart, brain and internal organs use protein as their primary building material. Protein even comprises a major portion of the blood and lymph, and is essential for proper hormone function and immune system health. Enough protein in the diet is absolutely essential in maintaining and building lean muscle tissue.

The primary role of dietary proteins is to supply amino acids for synthesis of the proteins required by the body. Amino acids are the building blocks the body uses to make its own unique proteins. In all organisms, proteins are constantly being synthesized and broken down. This process is called protein turnover. The average life of a protein molecule ranges from a few minutes to several weeks, depending on the kind of protein it is. Thus, the need for a continuous supply of good quality protein cannot be overemphasized.

In addition to being an essential nutrient for life, protein has a number of other specific benefits. Protein increases calcium absorption from the gut and preserves muscle and bone mass when one is dieting to lose weight. Protein promotes growth hormone release, which fosters fat burning and the preservation of lean body mass. Protein creates significantly more heat during metabolism than comparable amounts of carbohydrate. Most importantly, in terms of losing fat and changing body composition, protein is critical for building and repairing muscle tissue. When you are trying to lose fat, you reduce your calories. Unfortunately, your body views fat stores as more precious than your muscle tissue and will tend to burn up muscle tissue before it goes to fat for energy. This physiological adaptation, which at one time protected our ancestors from famine, no longer works in our favor. This is unfortunate, because muscle is our metabolically active tissue; it is our greatest calorie burner. Every action, from walking to breathing, and even blinking, is powered by muscle. The more muscle you have, the higher your metabolism and the more calories you burn, even at rest! Conversely, if you have less muscle mass, your metabolism will be slower. Pound for pound, muscle burns 25 times more calories than fat. One pound of muscle can burn 30 to 50 calories in a day, or 350 to 500 calories a week. One pound of fat only burns two calories a day or 14 in a week. *So, if you build just five pounds of muscle, that's equivalent to burning 26 pounds of fat in a year.* Therefore, building and preserving lean muscle tissue not only makes fat loss easier, but more permanent.

Muscle Weighs More Than Fat

Better measure of success – not the scale, but inches (fig.1).

Your Body = 100%
What is your body fat percentage or your ratio of muscle to fat?

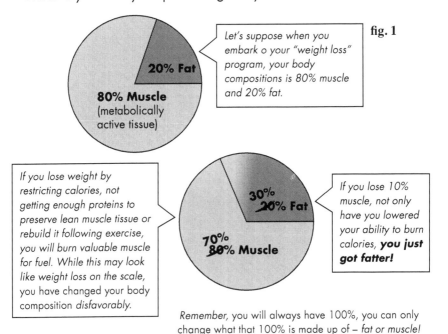

fig. 1

Let's suppose when you embark o your "weight loss" program, your body compositions is 80% muscle and 20% fat.

20% Fat

80% Muscle
(metabolically active tissue)

If you lose weight by restricting calories, not getting enough proteins to preserve lean muscle tissue or rebuild it following exercise, you will burn valuable muscle for fuel. While this may look like weight loss on the scale, you have changed your body composition *disfavorably.*

If you lose 10% muscle, not only have you lowered your ability to burn calories, **you just got fatter!**

30%
20% Fat

70%
80% Muscle

Remember, you will always have 100%, you can only change what that 100% is made up of – *fat or muscle!*

Eat more to weigh less?!

One of the best ways to ensure this muscle building, fat loss success is to consume small protein based meals throughout the day. Probably the biggest mistake people who are trying to lose body fat make, is to not eat enough. We think that by limiting calories, skipping meals, and not eating breakfast, we are certainly burning fat, right? Nothing could be more wrong. By eating only a couple of times a day, we slow down our metabolic rate as if we are putting our bodies into a state of fasting. This is actually store fat mode, rather than burn fat mode. What is worse is that our bodies will actually begin to catabolize, or burn, muscle tissue (not fat) for fuel. Yes, your body begins sacrificing brain tissue, internal organs, skin and muscle to supply you with the energy that you need to get through the day. Talk about self-defeating! Not only are you storing fat and permanently lowering your metabolism by breaking down precious muscle tissue, but if you are exercising to enhance your fat burning, body reshaping program, you are also depriving your body of the protein it needs to rebuild and repair what you have torn down in the gym.

Contrary to popular belief, you do not build muscle when you workout. Exercise, even weight lifting, actually breaks down muscle tissue creating an environment to *rebuild* it, stronger, firmer, toner. You need an adequate amount of protein in your diet, particularly immediately after working out, to recover and repair muscle tissue. This is critical for building and preserving lean muscle tissue. Without protein, your body must break down existing muscle to repair what was broken down in the gym. This is counter productive, and why so many people don't see the results they are looking for, and therefore become disillusioned with working out. Again, this is a common mistake that can be remedied by simply consuming an adequate amount of protein each and every day.

Keep the Fire Burning

Instead of trying to "not eat" to burn calories, we need to retrain ourselves to eat more frequently to stoke up our metabolism, and keep it burning in high gear. Think of your metabolism as a fire. Imagine you have just lit two fires. On one fire, toss a big, fat log on it, then, let it sit for several hours. On the second fire, you periodically feed chunks of firewood. Which fire is going to burn hotter and more efficiently? Obviously, the fire that you are constantly feeding with the right fuel burns better. When you return to the first fire, you'll find smoldering embers and half the log left unburned. Meanwhile, the second fire is hot enough to melt glass. Likewise, if we only eat a couple meals a day, particularly larger, heavier meals (because we are starving since we haven't eaten most of the day) we will end up with a sluggish, "smoldering" metabolism, and left over food or calories, stored as fat. On the other hand, if we feed our bodies small, frequent, protein based meals, not only will we keep our metabolism stoked and burning efficiently, we will be building and preserving that all important muscle tissue which will in turn further increase metabolism.

You will find that once you increase your protein intake, you will not only burn fat and see lean muscle gains faster, but you will recover from exercise faster, sleep better, have fewer cravings, and have TONS of energy!

A Few Words About Protein Quality

A **complete protein** contains all of the essential amino acids. Most animal proteins are complete, with the exception of gelatin, which is an incomplete animal protein as it is lacking in the essential amino acids tryptophan and tyrosine. An **incomplete protein** is one in which one or more of the essential amino acids are missing. Most plant proteins are incomplete, with the most notable exception being soybeans. Soybeans contain all essential amino acids making soy a complete plant protein. In fact, soy is a high quality complete protein that compares favorably with liver in amino acid composition. Incomplete proteins, no matter how ample the supply, cannot sustain animal life unless other proteins in the diet provide the missing amino acid or acids.

The *quality* of the protein in the diet is as important as the *quantity*. As much care should be devoted to choosing the quality of your protein as to getting enough quantity. Protein quality seems to be totally overlooked in today's official nutrition recommendations.

Protein Supplements – The Great Protein Shakedown
Shaking down what you've been shaking up.

So you get it. You've learned that protein is necessary to build and maintain lean muscle tissue, which is critical for maintaining or increasing metabolism. You've also learned that eating several times a day can also help preserve and build lean muscle tissue and increase metabolism. So supplementing protein once or twice throughout the day can certainly facilitate this process.

Sounds simple, right? Not so fast.

Just when you thought you've got it down, you're finding out that now you are faced with the task of choosing the RIGHT protein supplement. Not all protein products are created equal, in fact, some products marketed as protein shakes, actually contain very little protein and are loaded with sugar and/or fat...completely contrary to the goal you're trying to achieve.

So how do we begin to make a good choice?

First and foremost, when choosing a protein shake, or any supplement or food for that matter, **READ YOUR LABELS!** This is critical!

If you are choosing a prepackaged, pre-mixed product for convenience, make sure you choose one that at least uses a high quality protein source such as whey or soy, or a blend of whey, soy and casein. It also should'nt be loaded with sugar and fat. Many products claim to be "high in protein," but upon examination of the Nutrition Facts, we discover there is more than a 4 to 1 ratio of sugar to protein. There are products advertised to be a nutritious way to loose weight, high in protein and vitamins and now with heart healthy soy, that fail to mention the ingredient they are highest in -- *sugar!* With more than 42 grams of carbohydrates, 36 grams from sugar; that's equal to nine, yes NINE teaspoons, or 12 packets, of pure white sugar. I hardly see this as a "healthy" way to loose weight. It's more like a fast roller coaster ride through spikes in blood sugar and insulin, inconsistent energy levels and "yoyo" dieting. These are the very things that have led to the epidemic of obesity and diabetes. (More on this in the chapter on carbohydrates.) They also forget to mention the isoflavone content (the compounds that actually give soy all of its health benefits) of their soy product. Could it be because they are not actually in the product? A typical problem with soy products, now that they are realizing such popularity because of their health benefits, is that manufactures, for the sake of cost and flavor, are using cheaper sources of soy that have low or no isoflavones.

You also need to watch out for cheap drug store or discount store knockoffs of name brand protein products that, while they maintain their brand name, use less quantity and lower quality protein in a similar product made to look like their original higher quality product sold in health food stores. It's easy to get suckered at a large discount store or drugstore when you see a familiar brand name or packaging of a "reputable" product for a great price, only to find later that the price was "great" because the product actually has very little value. Many sports supplement companies that have been in the business for a long time and have gained reputation and name recognition, have ventured into the "quick buck from the masses who are suckers for weight loss products market." They have actually manufactured cheaper product look-a-likes containing extremely low quality proteins and flavored with cheaper ingredients, high in sugars and hidden saturated or trans saturated fats. Again, **READ YOUR LABELS!** The brand name and the package may not mean much.

Even label claims can be completely misleading. You would think a drink labeled for "low carb dieters" would be a fairly safe choice. Upon closer examination, you will find that in fact the carbs are low, (so is the protein quality for that matter), and if you don't mind 18 grams of fat from the #1 ingredient – CREAM, you are okay! I guess "for low carb, high fat dieters" would be a bit of an oxymoron, and "increases the risk of cardiovascular disease" wouldn't be a good selling point on the label.

Your best choice, to assure the highest quality in a protein, would be to choose a powdered product you mix yourself. You say "yuk – inconvenient and lumpy!" Wrong. Gone are the days where they are all clumpy, nasty tasting powders that must be mixed in the blender with all kinds of things added to cover the awful taste. A powder like ***OptiPRO M***® is a delicious protein that mixes easily in water, milk or any beverage with just a spoon or shaker. No mess, no clumps, no awful taste, just 100% high quality protein. And, with a product like this, you actually get more high quality protein, with other added nutrients and health benefits than the premixed shakes, and for less cost per serving – usually about $2 per "meal."

Be aware, however, that even within the world of protein powders, the quality levels differ drastically. Why does this matter? The lower the quality protein, the less bioavailable it is, or the less your body is able to absorb. Proteins, even within the same family, such as whey, may range in quality from *isolate* being the highest quality and the purest form, with the most biolavailibity, to *concentrate*, which is much less absorbable. Look for products that contain the isolate forms of whey and soy proteins. These are the highest quality and most bioavailable forms of two of the best protein sources for burning fat and building lean muscle tissue. Whey is very easily absorbed and is high in Branched Chained Amino Acids – critical to building muscle. Soy is high in the amino acids Glutamine and Arginine, which are essential to tissue repair, immune function and assist in fat loss and blood sugar regulation. Together they provide an optimized amino acid profile for fat loss and lean tissue gains. Soy also provides the additional benefits of antioxidant, anti carcinogenic protection, regulating cholesterol, promoting cardiovascular health, stabilizing blood sugar and balancing hormones in both men and women. Blending a high quality whey, which is very quickly digested, with another high quality, but slower digesting protein, will also provide you with the benefit of feeling fuller, longer.

Again, with blended products, not all proteins are created equally. **Beware of label loopholes!** A product may claim – (this is where the labels get misleading and confusing) to be 100% whey, and contain whey protein isolate …however, when you read the ingredients on the label, the first ingredient is some trademarked, proprietary name for the protein. Then, in parenthesis, you see a list of several different types of protein, including isolate. The parenthesis is the labeling loophole that allows the manufacturer to not list ingredients in the order of amount in the product. For example, whey protein isolate may be listed first within that parenthesis and whey protein concentrate last, however, the product could very well consist of 99% cheap protein concentrate or worse, hydrolyzed protein (gelatin – very unabsorbable) with no more than a sprinkling of isolate – just enough to list it on the label. You will find this on most of the large "value" size protein products – this explains their great "value." It's cheap to make a protein powder with hardly any protein in it. Also beware of exaggerated claims. Most claims on a certain product are not about that specific product at all, but refer to an ingredient, which might be common to all the other products, also. For example, "builds muscle 200 times faster;" 200 times faster than what? Any protein builds muscle 200 times faster than not eating at all.

Also, try to choose a protein supplement with added digestive enzymes. This will assure maximum absorbtion for maximum benefit, as well as help eliminate the digestive discomfort that is often associated with protein supplements.

So, Caveat Emptor! Or Let the Buyer Beware! Cheap and convenient don't always end up being best and usually not even cheap. Hopefully, armed with a little more information, you will be able to find a convenient cost effective protein product with what it takes to produce the results you are looking for. My best advice – Read your labels, be careful, do your homework, know if it sounds too good to be true it just might be. Always buy from a reputable source where you can be assured they stand behind the quality of their products. Be sure there is someone who can help you sort through claims, hype and misleading, confusing labels to assure you the highest quality, most cost effective product, that fits into your lifestyle and your goals.

Also, when choosing a protein food bar, choose wisely. Just like protein powders, not all bars claiming to be high protein/low carb are even close to what they claim. Stay away from bars with ingredients like hydrolyzed protein or gelatin. Not only are these forms of protein derived from bone marrow, hooves and beaks (YUK!), but they aren't proteins that your body can readily use. So why eat them?

Some Good Protein Choices

Chicken Breast (skinless/boneless, preferably Free Range, Hormone
     Free, NOT FRIED)

Turkey Breast --- preferably Free Range, Hormone Free

Lean ground turkey or beef --- preferably Free Range, Hormone Free

Eggs – Organic -- Whites or egg substitute

Fish – Always wild caught, NOT farm raised

    - Salmon (fresh or canned - packed in water, wild caught)

    - Tuna (fresh or canned - packed in water)

    - Orange Roughy

    - Tilapia

    - Mahi Mahi

    - Anchovies, Sardines

Ostrich -- Free Range, Hormone Free

Buffalo -- Free Range, Hormone Free

Crab, Lobster, Shrimp, Crawfish (can be low protein source for volume
     required)

Low-Fat Cottage Cheese

Soy Cheese

Vegetable Proteins – Soy products i.e.;

    - Tofu

    - Tempeh

    - Seitan

    - Veggie Burgers

Protein Shakes, Bars, Snacks

Carbohydrates

There are scarier things in this world than carbohydrates, like trans fats and MSG, but perhaps few that are less confusing. Good carbs, bad carbs, do I need carbs??? Let's try to get to the bottom of the carbohydrate question by arming ourselves with a little bit of knowledge. Be warned, you may have to read this chapter more than once before the light bulb goes off, but once you "get it," you will be able to take charge of the single most important thing that will produce the greatest, most broad ranging health benefits... your blood sugar.

Now for a quick "lesson" on carbohydrates. The most important thing to understand about carbohydrates is they have the most profound affect of ANY food on blood sugar and in turn, insulin, which collectively have the greatest affect on the most broad ranging health concerns, from body fat and cholesterol, to energy levels and restful sleep.

Carbohydrates are considered non-essential, meaning our bodies can manufacture the glucose normally obtained from eating carbohydrates. I know this sounds like we could eliminate them from our diet, but if we don't eat any carbohydrates, then our bodies will turn to muscle tissue for fuel. That's right, your body will burn those precious muscles for energy. And, since we now know that the amount of muscle tissue we have controls how fast or how slow our metabolism is, we don't want to lose muscle. For this reason, and because our brains don't work too well without them, we don't want to completely cut out carbs! We need them!

Carbohydrate foods consist mainly of glucose. When we consume and metabolize carbohydrates, our liver uses some of the glucose to replenish glycogen and sends the rest to our blood stream. When glucose enters the bloodstream, it stimulates the pancreas to secrete insulin. Insulin, in turn, regulates the level of glucose in the blood. Depending on the body's needs at the time, glucose may be converted to energy or stored as glycogen. If these actions do not lower blood glucose levels sufficiently, insulin will cause the excess glucose to be converted to fatty acids, and ultimately to body fat and cholesterol. The more insulin we have in our blood, the less we burn fat storages for energy and the more is stored, not only as body fat, but excess fatty acids are sent to your liver to be made into cholesterol. (fig. 2b)

Excessive consumption of carbohydrates in the form of sugar and starch is also a major factor in the development of high cholesterol (and atherosclerosis). However, if any carbohydrate foods could be singled out as important contributors to America's high blood cholesterol levels, they would have to be sucrose (or refined sugar) and high fructose corn sweeteners. both of which are composed of glucose and fructose. Once ingested, the glucose enters the bloodstream from which it is withdrawn by the cells and broken down by a series of reactions called glycolysis. Fructose also enters the bloodstream, but takes a different path. It bypasses the constraints imposed on the metabolism of glucose (glycolysis) and stimulated by the high insulin levels induced by the glucose component, moves directly to the biochemical pathway that makes cholesterol. In the early 1900's, when table sugar was a luxury, fruits were essentially the only source of fructose in the diet. When refined sugar became a prevalent part of every American diet, the consumption of fructose gradually increased. Later, the development and use of high fructose corn sweeteners in all sorts of commercial foods further added to the dietary burden of fructose. Today, fructose consumption is almost ten times that of two hundred years ago. As a result, it now accounts for a significant portion of the carbohydrate consumption in the American diet.

Dietary carbohydrates, and the metabolic hormone insulin, are the key agents in the synthesis and storage of body fat. It is a biochemical fact that excess blood glucose is ultimately converted to body fat. We have learned that a sure fire way to become overweight is to eat an excessive amount of carbohydrates, especially sugar, sweets and starches. Unfortunately, the major cause of today's epidemic of obesity is the result of overeating carbohydrate foods. Dietary fat and protein are not major factors in the cause of weight gain, obesity and the complications that go along with them.

So why am I supposed to eat carbs?! This is scary! Cholesterol, body fat, insulin increases?! Despite this frightening little lesson on carbohydrates, believe it or not, carbohydrates are still an important part of your diet. It's just important to choose the right ones. Carbohydrates act as important vehicles for countless micronutrients. Fruits and vegetables are a major source of fiber, minerals, vitamins A, C and E, and the only sources of important phytochemicals such as the carotenoids. When carbohydrates are very low in the diet, fats are used for energy, and proteins are used to supply the glucose needed for normal blood glucose levels. Carbohydrates are necessary to prevent the loss of muscle tissue.

The rate at which our blood stream absorbs glucose is called the **Glycemic Index.** Foods that cause a rapid rise in blood glucose levels have a high glycemic index and vice versa. (A list of these foods will be provided at the end of this section.) And why should I care about glycemic indices and all this carb mumbo jumbo? Well, studies have shown that high glycemic foods spike blood sugar, which in turn spike insulin levels, which ultimately doesn't satisfy hunger and can even increase your appetite. The rapid absorption of glucose from high glycemic foods induces a series of hormonal and metabolic changes that promote cravings, excessive food intake, poor energy levels and disrupted sleep.

High glycemic index foods, such as sugar and refined starches, also cause cortisol levels to rise. Cortisol is a hormone produced by the adrenal glands, and is usually associated with stress. However, it is not just stress that can elevate Cortisol levels; they are rapidly responsive to our food intake during each day. The glycemic index of a meal affects cortisol levels for up to the next five hours.

Why does this matter? Cortisol helps regulate many body functions including activation of thyroid hormone, muscle strength, energy production, resistance to infection and cancer, resistance to auto-immune diseases and intensity of allergic reactions. Cortisol is also a strong determinant in how rejuvenating sleep will be.

For individuals who start the day with a normal cortisol level, starchy or sugary breakfast food choices can cause the cortisol to overshoot the normal range. The cortisol will likely remain elevated all day – and all night, ultimately affecting weight management, energy levels and sleep. Worse than having a high glycemic meal is having no meal at all. A single late meal or skipped meal, within five hours of the previous meal or snack, tends to raise cortisol levels. A rise above the normal range during the day almost guarantees that the nighttime cortisol will be high, and thus disrupt REM sleep resulting in non-refreshing sleep. And don't forget, that skipped meal is also causing that precious, calorie burning muscle tissue to be burned for fuel.

Excess food intake and poor energy levels?! Who needs that?

To prevent the detrimental upward swing of cortisol and insulin, it's best to choose carbohydrate foods such as those from unprocessed, sprouted whole grains, green leafy and fibrous or cruciferous vegetables, nuts, beans and fruits and dairy products with low glycemic indices (a list of suggestions is included at the end of this chapter). It is also best to balance them with high quality protein foods. Foods high in sugars, refined carbohydrates and flours and starchy vegetables with high glycemic indices should be avoided when possible. Soft drinks and other sugary foods should be avoided or strictly limited. Proteins and fats have glycemic indices of zero, if they are not accompanied by carbohydrates. Complex carbohydrates, such as grains, beans and starches should be eaten in the earlier part of the day, and not as part of the dinner meal. It is best to include lots of green leafy, such as salad, and fibrous or cruciferous vegetables, such as broccoli or cabbage, with your lean protein for this meal.

By avoiding high glycemic foods, we can control the rate at which carbohydrates are converted to glucose and enter our bloodstream. Green leafy and fibrous vegetables, for example, especially when raw, are broken down slowly in the digestive system resulting in their carbohydrate content slowly being converted to glucose. In this case, blood glucose levels rise slowly, and the need for a quick and strong insulin response by the pancreas is minimized. This allows the pancreas to react slowly with a small amount of insulin and convert the glucose to glycogen, or fuel, which is the fuel needed to power our muscles and brains and even to burn fat *(see fig. 2a)*.

Blood Sugar and Insulin

Blood sugar and insulin should stay in close range.

key:	——— **Blood Sugar** - - - - **Insulin**

fig. 2a   When a balanced meal of proteins, carbs and fats is eaten, blood sugar rises slowly, insulin is secreted and blood glucose is converted by insulin to glycogen or energy.

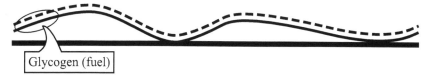

Glycogen (fuel)

A high-carbohydrate snack or meal, particularly one composed of sugar and/ or refined carbohydrates, triggers a series of events that lead a person down the road toward reactive hypoglycemia, fat storage and eventually diabetes. First, the carbohydrate snack is immediately converted to glucose, which causes a rapid rise in blood glucose. Second, the rapid rise in blood glucose prompts the pancreas to respond with secretion of an abnormally high level of insulin in an emergency-like attempt to keep blood glucose levels from rising too high. Third, within a short period of time, the excess insulin drives the blood glucose levels down to low or below normal levels *(see fig. 2b on page 28)*. The path that leads to reactive hypoglycemia is one that repeatedly follows this unhealthful dietary habit –satisfying hunger with high sugar/ starch snacks and soft drinks.

Blood Sugar and Insulin

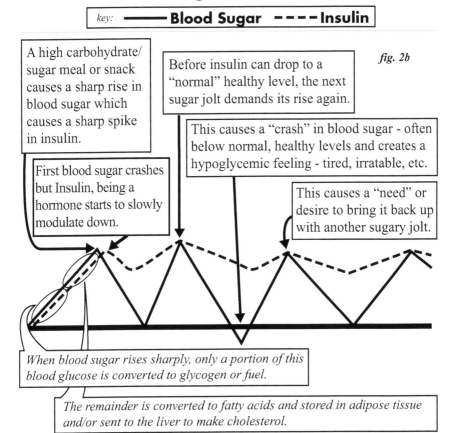

key: ——**Blood Sugar** – – – –**Insulin**

A high carbohydrate/ sugar meal or snack causes a sharp rise in blood sugar which causes a sharp spike in insulin.

Before insulin can drop to a "normal" healthy level, the next sugar jolt demands its rise again.

fig. 2b

This causes a "crash" in blood sugar - often below normal, healthy levels and creates a hypoglycemic feeling - tired, irratable, etc.

First blood sugar crashes but Insulin, being a hormone starts to slowly modulate down.

This causes a "need" or desire to bring it back up with another sugary jolt.

When blood sugar rises sharply, only a portion of this blood glucose is converted to glycogen or fuel.

The remainder is converted to fatty acids and stored in adipose tissue and/or sent to the liver to make cholesterol.

Why is this an unhealthful dietary habit? Because the high-carbohydrate snack, as explained above, causes a rapid rise in blood glucose followed by a rapid drop, which brings a feeling of hunger and weakness that demands another snack. The second snack relieves the symptoms briefly by supplying more glucose, but then restarts the hypoglycemic cycle with production of excess insulin. With time, this sort of dietary pattern can cause almost constant vague feelings of irritability, fatigue and general ill health. Repeatedly satisfying hunger with such foods leads to reactive hypoglycemia, and eventually, over a period of time, to insulin resistance (*see fig. 2c*).

Blood Sugar and Insulin

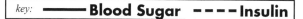

key: ———— **Blood Sugar** – – – – **Insulin**

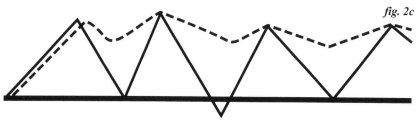

fig. 2c

*This constant rollercoaster of blood sugar levels and
continuously elevated insulin cause our cells to begin
to become insensitive to our own insulin. This is pre
diabetes - a.k.a. Metabolic Syndrome, Syndrome X.*

Reactive hypoglycemia, which is the proper name for hypoglycemia, is
more appropriately thought of as unstable blood sugar rather than low blood
sugar. Reactive hypoglycemia is a result of dietary habits that cause sharp
roller-coaster-like swings between very high blood glucose and very low
blood glucose. This can be prevented by avoiding snacks or meals that are
primarily sugars and refined starches such as pastries, cookies, cakes, donuts,
candy bars and soft drinks, even diet soft drinks. These products contain
mostly sugar and/or refined flour, both of which have high glycemic indices,
and are quickly converted to glucose. The use of artificial sweeteners is no
remedy. Certain artificial sugar substitutes, like sugar itself, also stimulate
the secretion of insulin. In fact, recent studies have shown that artificial
sugar substitutes might be more detrimental than sugar (we will discuss
sugar substitutes at greater length later in this chapter). As a result, these
foods cause a sharp rise in blood glucose levels. The pancreas receives a
high-glucose alarm from the sharp rise in blood glucose and quickly dumps
enough insulin into the blood to keep blood glucose levels under control.
Remember, not all carbohydrates have the same effect on blood glucose and
insulin levels. Refined grain products and sugar cause sharp rises in insulin
levels, but green vegetables and many fruits do not.

Reactive hypoglycemia does not occur in people who, in general, avoid refined carbohydrates and sugars in their diets. An occasional high-carbohydrate snack or meal will cause blood insulin levels to rise quickly to cope with the high blood glucose levels. Hunger and drowsiness will usually occur several hours after eating as the result of lowered blood glucose levels. However, because the pancreas is not abused by repeated unhealthy ingestion of high glycemic foods, it does not react with an excessive amount of insulin that remains in the blood long after it is needed.

Reactive hypoglycemia often leads to insulin resistance. Insulin resistance, as the term implies, is a resistance by the cells of the body to the presence of insulin. When insulin resistance occurs, the body's cells fail to permit insulin to transport glucose across their cell membranes. As a result, the cells become deficient in the glucose they need to function efficiently. Insulin resistance might be thought of as an inability on the part of cells to let insulin help them obtain the glucose they require. In healthy individuals, it is the sensitivity to insulin that allows glucose to be converted to glycogen and utilized by the cells of the body.

So how does hypoglycemia, or more precisely, unstable blood glucose, pave the way for insulin resistance? The up-and-down, roller-coaster swings in blood glucose concentration result in excessive secretion of insulin by the pancreas. With time, the mechanisms that enable cells to respond normally to insulin gradually become defective. Cells become exhausted and lose their sensitivity to insulin; they no longer utilize insulin the way they should. The lack of response by cells is *not* due to lack of insulin. The pancreas makes adequate amounts of insulin, but the cells just do not use it efficiently to metabolize glucose. As cells become more resistant to insulin, the fine-tuning of the relationship between blood glucose levels and the metabolic hormones, insulin and glucagons, is lost. The reduction in use of glucose by the cells and tissues of the body results in a gradual increase in the amount of glucose circulating in the blood. The high-low swings in blood glucose characteristic of hypoglycemia give way to longer periods of high blood glucose. This is termed hyperglycemia *(see fig. 2c)*.

Blood Sugar and Insulin

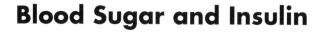

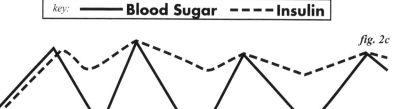

fig. 2c

This constant rollercoaster of blood sugar levels and continuously elevated insulin cause our cells to begin to become insensitive to our own insulin. This is pre diabetes - a.k.a. Metabolic Syndrome, Syndrome X.

The most obvious symptoms of insulin resistance are weight gain and feelings of fatigue and weakness that are sometimes overwhelming. The feelings of fatigue and weakness are due to what might be called cellular starvation. Cells and tissues cannot transfer sufficient glucose into themselves to provide the energy they require to function properly. Overwhelming fatigue and weight gain results.

Along with the hyperglycemia that eventually results from insulin resistance come serious, long-term damaging effects. Insulin resistance is associated with high blood pressure, obesity, high blood levels of triglycerides and LDL (bad) cholesterol, low blood levels of HDL (good) cholesterol, contribute to the aging process, and are thought to promote degenerative diseases such as Alzheimer's disease.

Diabetes, disease or bad habit?

When the discussion of blood sugar or diabetes comes up, I often hear "diabetes runs in my family". My response to that is often "the bad habits that cause diabetes run in your family." Despite differences in susceptibility to type-2 diabetes, there is strong clinical and epidemiological evidence that the underlying cause is consumption of excessive sugar and refined carbohydrates. The good news is, since diet is the cause, diet can be the solution to reversing it.

The connection between type-2 diabetes and obesity is insulin resistance. As described above, repeated large releases of insulin into the bloodstream in response to high blood glucose levels cause the body's cells to become resistant to the stimulus of insulin. When this happens, the pancreas must secrete larger and larger amounts of insulin in an attempt to lower glucose. Fat cells do not become as resistant to insulin as do other body cells; hence, the deposition of fat that is stimulated by insulin continues after other body cells become resistant.

Despite increased secretion of insulin, blood glucose levels rise above normal levels because cells and tissues of the body are not able to remove glucose efficiently from the blood. Eventually, the pancreas becomes exhausted and reaches its insulin production limit. This allows blood glucose levels to rise to unsafe levels, despite futile attempts by the pancreas to secrete sufficient insulin to lower them. The result is type-2 diabetes, also known as adult-onset diabetes or noninsulin dependent diabetes mellitus (NIDDM) *(see fig. 2d on pg 33)*.

Blood Sugar and Insulin

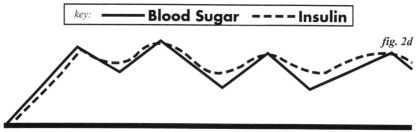

When blood sugar can no longer be converted to glucogen by insulin, blood sugar levels remain high. This is diabetes.

The good news is that the path that leads to a return to a normal insulin/blood sugar balance is a simple one to follow, and the same one that leads to better energy levels, fewer cravings, better weight management, better sleep, better cardiovascular health, better brain function and better overall health. It is the path to true vitality, and one that starts with frequent small meals and snacks that are protein based and balanced to include whole grains, fibrous carbohydrates from vegetables and good fats.

We need a minimum of 20% and a maximum of 40% of our diet to come from carbohydrates, and growing children and active adults need more carbohydrates than older or sedentary people. (See General Guidelines and Guidelines for Caloric Breakdown before sample menus.)

A word about
Artificial vs. All Natural Sweeteners

I know, you may be thinking, "I've been told to cut out refined sugar from my diet, but please don't tell me I can't have artificial sweeteners either! What about my diet Cokes? Splenda in my iced tea?" Well, consider this to be more of an informational piece; you draw your own conclusions.

Artificial Sweeteners

We've all heard the rumors: Sweet-n-Low causes cancer! Nutra-Sweet will give you seizures! But how much of this is true? First, I would recommend that everyone stay away from aspartame, a.k.a. NutraSweet and Equal. Aspartame has been directly correlated to neurological disorders. There have been numerous scholarly articles and books written by doctors and scientists on the dangerous effects aspartame has on the brain. If you're in a pinch and you absolutely must have that diet drink, choose one that doesn't use aspartame, such as diet Coke with Splenda. Saccharin or Sweet-n-Low should also be avoided if at all possible, but it is not as dangerous as aspartame. Thirdly, there's the artificial sweetener sucralose or Splenda, which is the lesser of the three evils. Sucralose is sugar chemically modified by replacing the glucose molecules with chlorine molecules. Although we come in contact with chlorine in our tap water and showers, it is not recommended that we ingest any more than we already do. When choosing a sweetener, your best bet is to go with an all natural one.

All Natural Sweeteners

Although all natural sweeteners don't pose any health risks, they can sometimes be difficult to handle. Stevia, for instance, is an all natural, plant derived sweetener that is 200-300 times sweeter than sugar. And while a little bit can go a long way, it is difficult if not impossible to use in your recipes. Also, because it is an herb, some stevia products can be sweeter/more bitter than others. Stevia also changes its potency over time, resulting in a bitter taste if let to sit for too long in that pitcher of iced tea or cup of coffee. Other all natural sweeteners that have gained popularity are the sugar alcohols: xylitol, maltitol, sorbitol, etc. The plus side to sugar alcohols is that they are great for diabetics because they can't permeate the walls of the intestines, therefore making it impossible for them to adversely affect one's blood sugar levels. The down side, however, is that because sugar alcohols can't permeate the intestinal walls, they have a low laxation threshold. This means that they can cause a laxative effect or gastrointestinal discomfort. Also, sugar alcohols have ⅔ the calories of sugar. You might as well use sugar! So what is the solution? Finally, there is an all natural Sweetener, Swerve™, that is as close to sugar as it gets, with zero calories and zero glycemic index. Swerve™ looks, tastes, measures, cooks, bakes, candies and even freezes like sugar. Yes, now you can bake your cake and eat it too! Your favorite indulgences are no longer a "no no" as they can be made over to be lower calorie, healthier options. Swerve™ is made from the fibrous parts of fruits and vegetables, through a natural enzyme process that actually yields white crystals. This means NO chemical processing of any kind. And, with zero calories and zero glycemic index there is no rise in blood sugar or insulin, making it perfect for diabetics and everyone wanting to watch their weight and better their health. And because Swerve™ is 100% as sweet as sugar, its easy to measure when substituting in cooking and baking. Swerve™ also has a high digestive tolerance (no gas and bloating. . .or worse) and provides prebiotic activity to foster friendly flora in your gut for better digestion. Swerve™ is the perfect sugar alternative and is unlike anything out there!

Carbohydrates

The following are examples of simple carbohydrates:

Sugars

Fructose (fruit), Lactose (dairy), Dextrose, Sucrose (sugar)

Fruits

There are good and bad choices in the world of simple carbohydrates. The trick is to make good simple carb choices. Try eliminating refined sugars and choosing low glycemic fruits. Also, try replacing breads or carbs with apples, celery or carrots for dips or spreads. These are carbohydrate foods that will satisfy your carb cravings and provide you with fiber, vitamins and nutrients. Below is a list of other fruits and veggies to add to your diet.

Choose fruits that are colorful for their antioxidant quality.

Berries – Acaí, Blueberries (best choice followed by other berries)	Cranberries
	Grapefruit
Strawberries	Guava
Blackberries	Kiwi
Raspberries	Lemon
Goji Berries	Lime
Pomegranate	Orange
Red Grapes (eat seeds – high in nutritional value)	Papaya
	Peach
Cherries (Bing or Dark with pits)	Plum
Apples (granny smith are best)	Tangerine
Cantaloupe	*Limit bananas

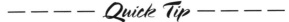

— — — — *Quick Tip* — — — —

If you want to add bananas to your smoothie, peel and cut a ripe banana into quarters and freeze. Using a quarter of a very ripe frozen banana will add taste and texture without all of the sugar.
Frozen berries make the best addition to your smoothie.

Vegetables (Fibrous)

The following are great choices. They are full of fiber and should be included with lunch and dinner.

Asparagus	Mustard Greens
Broccoli	Okra
Brussels Sprout	Onion
Cabbage	Parsley
Cauliflower	Peppers-Red and Yellow Bell Peppers
Celery	Pumpkin
Cucumber	Radish
Chives	Spinach
Collards	String Beans
Eggplant	Squash – Spaghetti and Acorn
Endive	Tomato
Kale	Turnip
Leeks	Zucchini
Lettuce	

No peas or corn and limit carrots

Carbohydrates (Complex)*
Brown Rice
Oatmeal
Sweet potatoes
Whole Grain Breads (sprouted wheat, Ezekiel)
Brown rice pasta

Consume in A.M. and at lunch, limit at night.

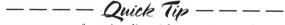

— — — — *Quick Tip* — — — —

Try some Hummus or your favorite dip with carrots or celery sticks instead of chips to save calories, carbs and get those servings of veggies in.

Fats and Essential Fatty Acids

The wonderful world of fats and oh, how we need them. While protein is the most important macronutrient you can eat, fats are undeniably essential for countless bodily functions. Fats, or essential fatty acids (EFAs), which include omega-3s, 6s and 9s, are exactly that: essential. This means your body cannot manufacture these fats so they must be supplied through the diet. Without fats, the body cannot absorb the fat soluble vitamins A, D, E and K. Fats are also needed for proper brain function, joint mobility, cardiovascular health (yes, some fats are good for your heart), and the production of prostaglandins or hormone-like substances that regulate many bodily functions. Essential fatty acids are also necessary for burning fat. But this doesn't mean you should go out and buy a block of cheese and start slicing! One must know the difference between good fats and bad fats.

When deciding on what kinds of fats to cut back on, you want to limit saturated fats that come from animal fats like creams, cheeses and butter, and try to eliminate trans fats completely from your diet. However, it is probably safer and better for you to consume a saturated fat like butter than a hydrogenated fat like "traditional" margarine, which is often almost all hydrogenated oil. You can also look for brands like Smart Balance or Earth Balance, which are "buttery spreads" that contain no trans fats and are actually high in EFAs. Read your labels! Avoid products that contain hydrogenated oils, partially hydrogenated oils or monoglycerides. These are all trans fatty acids. Also, don't just look at the Nutrition Facts panel that may state zero trans fats. You may be fooled by the old portion size loophole trick! Always look at the ingredients statement to see if these words show up. If so, you don't want it. Hydrogenated oils, or trans fats, are oils that have been subjected to high temperatures, extreme pressure, and the addition of extra hydrogen atoms. This process extends the shelf life of many food products. But what does this have to do with my body? A lot. First, trans fats cannot be digested by the body or utilized in any way. Also, hydrogenated oils have been linked with increased risk of heart disease, type II diabetes, high cholesterol and breast cancer in women. Trans fats are most commonly found in margarine, some cookies and crackers, candy bars and many frying oils. Since these fats are basically unusable by your body, and, in fact, can be potentially harmful, why put them in your body?

Essential Fatty Acids

While many of us have heard of essential fatty acids (EFAs), we may not quite understand how they are useful to us, or how to choose good sources of them. A growing body of research shows that long chain fatty acids, or omega-3 in fish, flaxseed, oils and fish oil supplements, lower most of the major cardiovascular risk factors, including high blood pressure, sticky platelets in the blood that may form clots in the arteries, and high triglycerides linked to both heart disease and insulin resistance. Omega-3 fats also help the heart beat in a regular rhythm, while preventing leakage and swelling of the blood vessels. In addition, several studies suggest that omega-3 supplements help reduce the risk of colon cancer, and other evidence indicates that these fats may slow the rate of metastasis in breast cancer.

Rich in beneficial omega-3 fats, salmon has become a staple of healthy eating. It is important, however, to know whether salmon is caught in the wild or farmed in ocean tanks. These farms are often viewed as hog lots or feedlots of the ocean. Farmed fish breed disease and parasites and have come under scrutiny for not only causing pollution, but also endangering wild stock. More importantly, researchers have found that farm raised salmon have 10 times the levels of polychlorinated biphenyls (PCBs) than wild caught. Linked to both breast cancer and non-Hodgkin's lymphoma, PCBs also appear to cause irreversible brain damage in the developing fetus. The U.S. Department of Agriculture (USDA) has also discovered that farmed salmon contains more than twice the saturated fats and fewer omega-3 fatty acids than wild salmon. In fact, the white lines running through its flesh is fat from the feed stock, and the pink color is from dye in the feed stock, rather than the natural "salmon" color of the wild caught fish. Fish caught in the wild aquire this color because of the high levels of the potent antioxidant carotinoid, astaxanthin from their largely vegetarian diet of algae. Also, because wild caught salmon have a shorter life span they are less likely to accumulate toxins.

Besides salmon, fish that contain 5% or more of the healthy fats include:

Albacore tuna	Mackerel
Bluefin tuna	Sablefish (black cod)
Anchovies	Sardines
Herring	Trout

Fish that offer between 2.5 and 5% omega-3 fatty acids include:

Atlantic halibut	Swordfish
Bluefish	Yellowfin tuna
Mullet	

Fish with less than 2.5% of these fats, but are still beneficial include:

Cod	Red snapper
Croaker	Rockfish
Flounder	Sea bass
Grouper	Shark
Haddock	Sole
Pacific halibut	Whiting
Pollock	

Food Alone is Not Enough

Essential means we need them, and because it's difficult to get an adequate amount of Essential Fatty Acids in our diet, it is necessary to supplement them. There are two groups of essential fatty acids, the omega-3 group and the omega-6 group. These essential fatty acids are the key building blocks for brain, nerve and eye tissue, as well as the starting materials for a large group of hormone-like messenger biochemicals, known as eicosanoids, that regulate dozens of vital life functions.

One source of these essential fats, flax oil, has become increasingly popular. Flax is high in Omega-3 fatty acids and is great for it's high lignan and high fiber content. Lignans are compounds found in plants, and are one of the two major classes of phytoestrogens, which are important because they may help prevent estrogen dependent cancers, including prostate cancer in men. Flax, however, is made of omega-3's from ALA (Alpha Linoleic Acid), which is not readily convert to EPA (Eicosapentaenoic Acid) and DHA (Docosahexaenoic Acid). This does not make it the best source of necessary omega-3's. Substances like trans fats can further disrupt this process.

EPA, alone or with other omega-3 sources, has been shown to be effective in a number of conditions, most of which involve its ability to lower inflammation. Omega-3 fatty acids, in particular EPA, is thought to possess beneficial potential in certain mental conditions.

DHA is an omega-3 essential fatty acid, and is the primary building block of the central nervous system, as well as every cell in the body. It is also metabolized to form several families of potent hormones. DHA is a major fatty acid in sperm and brain phospholipids, and especially in the retina. Dietary DHA can reduce the level of blood triglycerides in humans, which may reduce the risk of heart disease. Low levels of DHA result in reduction of brain serotonin levels and have been associated with ADHD, Alzheimer's disease and depression, among other diseases. There is mounting evidence that DHA supplementation may be effective in combating such diseases. DHA is also a critically important supplement for pregnant and nursing mothers. In the first trimester of pregnancy, the fetal brain doubles in size and the eyes begin to develop, making it critical that expectant mothers have sufficient stores of omega-rich fats. Nursing mothers also pass DHA on to their infants via breast milk, only to have their own stores further depleted. Without supplementation, this drain of DHA reserves is considered a contributing factor in postpartum depression.

The easiest way to ensure you are getting enough of the omega-3's DHA, essential for brain function, mood and focus, and EPA, essential for cardiovascular health and joint mobility, is take a high quality fish oil supplement. This is very important. I know, it doesn't sound appetizing, however, fish oils are available in a gel cap form or as a liquid. Believe it or not, the liquid fish oils don't taste nearly as bad as you may think. Always look for oils that are pharmaceutical grade, highly molecularly distilled, are free of heavy metals and PCBs, and are packaged under nitrogen in dark bottles. The nitrogen flush is critically important to ensure the oils don't oxidize or turn rancid. Rancid oils are actually detrimental to your health and have been shown to be carcinogenic. Bad omega-3 oils are worse that no oils at all. The best way to ensure you are taking a quality product is to always purchase your oils from a reputable health food store and look for oils from reputable companies like Nordic Naturals or Wellness Innovations. Vegetarians wishing to benefit from these same omega 3's as fish, not from an animal source, may choose algae-based supplements, such as Neuromins.

To get the best of both the worlds of fish and flax, I recommend taking a liquid fish oil supplement once daily, and using flax in the form of ground flax, added to your shakes or sprinkled on salads and cereals. This way you are certain to get the DHA and EPA necessary for brain function, mood and focus, cardiovascular health and joint mobility, as well as the lignans and fiber flax has to offer.

Omega-6 fatty acids, which are also essential, should not be neglected, and should come from sources not damaged in processing. Good sources of these polyunsaturated fats include herbs like borage and evening primrose oil, nuts and seeds. The body converts omega-6s into prostaglandins, hormone like substances vital in controlling the circulatory system, heart function, healthy skin, and immune function. An inadequate or unbalanced supply of omega-3 and omega-6 fatty acids may actually cause inflammation and associated disease, such as heart attacks, high blood pressure, asthma, arthritis, infertility, migraines and more.

These fatty acids, and the balance of them, are strongly related to both health and disease. Beneficial health effects are found when diets contain adequate levels of both, with a low ratio of omega-6 to omega-3, optimumly between a 4 to 1 and a 1 to 1 ratio. But, because our American diet is so high in Omega-6s, and we rarely adequately supplement omega-3s, we often end up with an imbalance of eicosanoids, those biochemicals that regulate so many vital functions, and the detrimental effects, such as inflammation, cardiovascular disease, hypertension, diabetes, obesity and cancer. To ensure a good balance, supplement with at least 2 grams of omega-3s daily. If additional omega-6s are recommended for specific health conditions, such as skin or hormones, be certain to increase omega-3 supplementation to maintain balance.

A Word About Cooking Oils

How oils are processed and the smoke point of various fats are important to note when choosing your favorite fat for cooking. Be certain that you select oil that is expeller pressed, or organic, to be certain it is free of harmful petrochemical solvents.

Smoke points are also important, as it is believed that fats that have gone past their smoke points contain a large quantity of free radicals which contribute to the risk of cancer. Once a fat starts to smoke, it has begun to break down and is no longer good for consumption.

Canola Oil

Canola oil is widely, and erroneously, recognized as the healthiest salad and cooking oil available. It is made through hybridization of rapeseed, and the oil is removed by a combination of high temperature mechanical pressing and solvent extraction. Traces of the solvent (usually hexane) remain in the oil, even after considerable refining. Obviously this is not the best choice!

Olive Oil

Extra-virgin olive oil is an excellent source of monounsaturated fats, good fats that may lower the risk of heart disease. It has a low smoke point of 250 degrees. Because of this, it is not the best for cooking. Use olive oil after cooking a dish for flavor or in salad dressings.

Use plain olive oil (smoke point 450 Degrees) for cooking.

Grape-Seed Oil

It's 420 degree smoke point makes grape-seed oil great for cooking over high heat. It also emulsifies well, making it easy to whip into mayonnaise.

Avocado Oil

This oil has an exceptionally high smoke point of 500 degrees, making it the best and safest choice for sautéing and pan frying.

MCTs: Medium Chain Triglycerides & Tropical Oils

There is a category of saturated fats that are actually good for you. These fats come from the tropical oil family. Coconut oil, believed in the 1980s to be harmful like all other saturated fats, can truly be part of a healthy diet. The saturated fat in coconut oil is lower in calories than animal fats and vegetable oils. It is also identical to a special group of fats found in human breast milk called medium-chain triglycerides (MCTs). Unlike long-chain fatty acids, which are repackaged by the body and stored in fat cells, MCTs are sent straight to the liver and converted into energy. In this respect, MCTs act more like carbohydrates than fats. Coconut oil also has a high post meal metabolic boost, which means you burn more calories. Consuming coconut oil will help give you more energy, make you feel fuller, stimulate thyroid activity and normalize cholesterol levels by converting LDL into vital anti-plaque hormones. If that's not enough of a good thing, coconut oil is about 50% lauric acid, which is a beneficial fatty acid also found in abundance in human breast milk. Lauric acid is anti-viral, antibacterial, antiprotozoal, and is used by the body to destroy viruses, various bacteria and protozoa.

Coconut oil also consists of Caprylic acid, which has antimicrobial and yeast killing properties. Coconut oil fat also normalizes body lipids, protects against alcohol damage in the liver and improves the immune system's anti-inflammatory response.

Coconut oil also possesses numerous antioxidant properties. Its natural antioxidants, and resistance to change from heat, give coconut oil a long shelf life (over a year without refrigeration) and make it ideal for cooking and baking. Try substituting coconut oil for butter or canola oil in your favorite cookie, brownie or cake recipe for a lower calorie healthier treat.

CLA: Conjugated Linoleic Acid

What if there was a fat that could burn fat, preserve and build lean muscle tissue and inhibit future fat storage, all while delivering other critical health benefits like promoting healthy blood sugar and cholesterol levels, enhancing immune function and providing powerful anti-inflammatory and antioxidant protection? We'll there is – CLA or conjugated linoleic acid. This remarkable fatty acid is a fat that burns fat and preserves lean muscle tissue. It actually prevents fats from being deposited into cells. The less fat that is present in the cells, the smaller and less mature they become; this helps to reduce the level of fat in the body. CLA also works to increase lean muscle mass by enhancing the enzyme activity in muscle cells. The increased presence of fat will be burned in the muscle cells, thus building up lean muscle mass.

Many times, when one begins a diet, he or she may lose fat, but they are also losing valuable muscle tissue. They essentially become a smaller version of their older self or "skinny fat." Pound for pound, muscle tissue burns, on average, five times more calories than fat. This is why it is so important to maintain lean muscle tissue. Now, with CLA, you can lose the fat, but not the muscle. This is certainly a more effective way to combat fat and beat the effects of "yo-yo" dieting. Rather than just restricting calories, which ultimately results in loss of our metabolically active calorie-burning muscle tissue, CLA helps accomplish your real goal of a true change in body composition. But don't jump on the scale to measure you results. Muscle weighs three times what fat does, so a positive change in body composition can look misleadingly disappointing on the scale. With CLA you can see the inches disappear, particularly in that stubborn abdominal region, so it's important to choose a better measure of success. Find that pair of jeans you just can't quite zip, or that favorite suit that now lives in the back of your closet, and let those, or the notches in your belt, be your true measures of success.

It is important to note that, not all products that claim to be or have CLA in their formulas are created equally. There are only two companies in the world that have rights to the patented form of CLA. The University of Wisconsin Alumna Research Foundation owns the patents on the manufacturing process for CLA, and has given the rights to use this patented process to two companies – Clarinol and Tonalin. OptiCLA® by PhytoCeutical Formulations, LLC is currently the only product on the market that is a powdered CLA in triglyceride form, the way it occurs naturally in food. OptiCLA® provides the full 4.6 grams, clinically shown to provide all the fat burning and other health benefits, in each serving. The CLA products in a capsule form are the free fatty acid form of CLA, which is hard to digest and has often been associated with stomach upset. Additionally, each 1000mg capsule nets an average of 72% - 84% CLA, which means you would have to take 8-10 of these pills a day to get the efficacious dose. Not only is this difficult to do, but it can also become very expensive. With OptiCLA® by PhytoCeutical Formulations, the full daily dose can easily be mixed into a protein shake or other beverage, or added to food, providing the optimal fat burning, lean tissue building dose in just one scoop, once a day.

Naturally you may ask, "Can I get CLA in my food?" Although CLA is a naturally occurring component of the human diet, it occurs at concentrations far too small to deliver weight management and other health benefits. In the US, for example, with the trend towards a diet low in fats and increased use demonstrated at dosages of 3.5 grams to 6 grams per day. Achieving this level requires supplementation.

While CLA has been getting most of its accolades through its effects on weight loss, this remarkable fat has also been putting its mark on many other broad ranging health concerns from blood sugar and cholesterol to inflammation, cancer and overall immunity. CLA was actually discovered as the compound that naturally occurred in meat, that inhibited tumor metastasis in breast cancer, and may also be protective against colon cancer. Supplementation with CLA has also been shown to stimulate immune response against the influenza virus and hepatitis B by increasing the presence of virus specific antibodies.

CLA is certainly the one and only fat burner that has so many overwhelming health benefits; it's easy to consider it as a recommended daily supplement.

Fats

⅛ cup (2 TBL) roasted/raw/unsalted of the following:

> Peanuts (approx. 10-12 nuts)
>
> Almonds (approx. 8-10 nuts)
>
> Cashews (approx. 12 nuts)
>
> Walnuts (approx. 5-6 nuts)
>
> Pecans (approx. 8 nuts)
>
> Brazil Nuts (approx. 3-4 nuts)
>
> Soynuts (⅓ cup) – also good source of protein
>
> Pumpkin Seeds

Nut Butter – 1 TBL Unsalted Peanut, Almond or Soy

Avocado – Half

Olives - 10

Olive Oil – 1 TBL

Coconut Oil

CLA

Flax Oil – good source of Omega 3 Fatty Acids

*Fish – good sources of Omega 3 Fatty Acids:

> Tuna (6 oz)   Sardines
>
> Salmon (6 oz)   Mackerel
>
> Anchovies

*When these are used as Protein source, they also count as a Fat source.

Why Exercise -

What kind and how much?
Cardio vs. Weight Training

While it may feel like running on the treadmill for an hour (while you are dripping with sweat) is burning tons of calories, it's only burning calories while you are exercising and for one to two hours after. If you really want to lose fat – and keep it off -- the best way to do it is with weight training. Weight training is the single most effective way to permanently increase your metabolism. The more muscle you have, the more fat you burn all the time – 24hours a day, 7 days a week -- not just one or two hours when you're exercising, but every hour of every day, whether you're exercising, eating, sleeping or sitting at your desk. Pound for pound, muscle burns 25 times more calories than fat. One pound of muscle can burn 30 to 50 calories in a day, or 350 to 500 calories a week. One pound of fat only burns two a day or 14 in a week. So, if you build just five pounds of muscle, that's equivalent to burning 26 pounds of fat in a year.

The evidence is right in front of you in the gym.

Notice the number of overweight people who do hours of cardio on the treadmill, in aerobics classes or on the bike – or worse, all of the above. The same people, on the same program for months, maybe even years, with no noticeable results. Then, compare them to the physiques in the weight room. Ask some of those people who look the most fit how much time they really spend in the gym – it's much less than you think. The results produced by weight training are much more effective. If your own research isn't convincing enough to back up these claims, consider a Tufts University study that showed strength and resistance training can increase metabolism by seven percent, and promote significant changes in body composition. Scientists calculated the higher metabolic rate meant that resistance trained subjects burned an average of an extra 354 calories per day. The final result was that weight training produces an increase in lean body mass and a decrease in body fat by a permanent increase in metabolic rate.

What about the scale?

Throw it out! Yes, you may end up weighing the same or even more because muscle weighs more than fat, but remember, muscle takes up less space than fat. So ultimately, you will be smaller, firmer and more toned…and your clothes will fit better. That's the true test, how you look and how you feel – not what the numbers on the scale say. And women do not become overly muscular. It's just not possible – women don't naturally produce enough of the hormones it takes to grow massive muscle. Weight training will, however, give you that tone look you're striving for – you can't burn fat off to see muscle tone that doesn't exist. In addition, weight training is important to help prevent osteoporosis by building and maintaining bone density.

Timing is everything.

If your primary goal for cardio, in addition to cardio vascular health, is to burn fat, the most effective time to do it is when glycogen stores are low, therefore, early morning on an empty stomach would be an optimum time since glycogen stores have been depleted throughout the night while you slept.

If morning isn't an option, and you'll be doing cardio in the same workout session as weight training, it's better to do cardiovascular activity immediately following weight training because glycogen levels have also been depleted at this time. Not only will your cardiovascular exercise be more effective at fat burning, but your weight training session will be more effective and intense since you won't have burned up all your ATP on cardio.

The key to successful weight loss is balance – in both diet and exercise. Weight training will help increase lean body composition and boost your metabolism, even while at rest. While cardiovascular activity will help muscles utilize oxygen more efficiently and promote overall good cardiovascular health. Remember though, too much cardio can actually burn valuable muscle tissue, and losing muscle slows down your metabolism -- which is obviously counter productive to your whole weight loss goal. Again, remember balance -- allow your body time to recover from all exercise. Muscle tissue needs recovery time to repair and grow. So don't be afraid to take a couple of days off with no exercise, and you will actually see better results.

Why Supplements?

The Case for Supplementation

"Do you believe in supplements?" It's a question often asked as if taking vitamins were based on some kind of blind faith that they will actually provide some benefit or serve some useful purpose. Thankfully supplementation, as a progressive and proactive approach to healthcare, is not based on blind faith, but on a growing body of science that is finally taking its place alongside other health sciences. What I do believe is that more and more people are increasingly interested in nutrition as a means of improving their lives and preventing illness. They want to live longer, healthier lives, look better, feel better, handle stress better, have more energy and minimize their risk of everything from the common cold to cancer.

As Americans seek to attain longer, healthier lives, and to reduce chronic disease, the evidence to encourage the use of supplements grows stronger. A recent study commissioned by the Council for Responsible Nutrition estimated that 8.7 billion dollars could be saved on four major diseases if Americans consumed optimum levels of the antioxidants vitamin C, vitamin E, and beta-carotene. Diets optimal in these nutrients have been shown to reduce costs associated with breast, lung and stomach cancer, and dramatically reduce the incidence and severity of cataracts. Additionally, the council evaluated ten years of the best scientific studies related to the benefits of vitamin and mineral supplements and concluded that the long term benefits could reduce neural tube birth defects by 70 percent, sick days could be reduced by 50 percent and health-care costs by delaying cardiovascular disease, stroke and hip fracture could be reduced by a staggering $89 billion per year.

And while perhaps some of these benefits could be derived from diet, most individuals do not eat the five servings of fruit and vegetables as recommended by the National Cancer Institute. In fact, it has been estimated that less than 10 percent of Americans actually consume two servings of fruit and three servings of vegetables per day, and that over half eat no vegetables at all. As for those of us who do practice better eating habits, and do include those daily five, we are still being left nutritionally void of many of the nutrients we believe we are consuming.

Food is not what it used to be.

Today our food is both less (nutritionally speaking) and more (chemically contaminated) than in the past. On an average our food travels 1300 miles from farm to market shelf. Nearly every state buys 90 percent of its food from out of the state. Through irradiation, our food is bombarded with the equivalent of 233 billion chest x-rays to kill bacteria and extend shelf life. Thirty percent of American dairy animals are fed genetically engineered bovine growth hormone.

Many modern agricultural practices adversely affect the quality of our food and its nutrient levels. Many foods are grown using methods designed to increase quantity or to facilitate transportation and storage, and these methods often are detrimental to the nutritional value of the food. Modern farming methods also often degrade the quality of the soil in which our food is grown leaving it very low in minerals, and with added pesticides, herbicides and other chemicals that are added during the growing process. High nitrogen fertilizers accelerate growth so fruits and vegetables are marketable size, long before they have had time to absorb minerals or synthesize nutrients. Often foods are not allowed to develop to their full level of vitamins and minerals, which increases greatly during later stages of growth. Fruits and vegetables are often picked before they are ripe, or allowed to ripen during transit to the market, which greatly diminishes their vitamin or mineral content. Transportation and storage can also adversely affect nutrient content of fruits and vegetables as they can start to lose significant amounts of vitamins as soon as they are cut or harvested. Transit time alone can provide for produce that has been severely depleted of its nutrient content. Produce can lose as much as 50 percent of its carotene (pro-vitamin A) and 60 percent of its vitamin C within as little as three days of being harvested. Additionally, certain fruits and vegetables can lose significant amounts of vitamins when they are stored at cold temperatures or even at room temperatures. Green vegetables lose all of their vitamin C after just a few days of being stored at room temperature. Drying, as well as exposure to light and oxygen also diminishes nutrient content. And while some may argue that many foods have been grown with the addition of certain nutrients, the nutrients optimum for plant growth are not necessarily optimum for our consumption. Chemical fertilizers that facilitate plant growth do not replace the minerals necessary for human nutrition. Even organic fruits and vegetables, while they are free of pesticides, are still harvested and transported using these same practices, unfortunately also rendering them nutritionally insufficient. And unfortunately, produce is not the only food group fallen victim to modern processing and refining practices. Whole grains have suffered probably the greatest injustice inflicted by the food industry. When wheat is processed in to white flour, up to 40 percent of the vitamin C, 65-85 percent of the various B Vitamins, 59 percent of the magnesium and 72 percent of the zinc are lost along with significant amounts of protein and fiber. All in all, more than 26 essential nutrients are removed. Even our meat, fish and dairy products do not contain the nutrients we assume they do.

Supplements are a way for us to make up for nutrients lost in our food as a result of growing, shipping, storing and processing practices. Incorporating a good multivitamin into your daily routine is a good start to optimizing your nutrition plan, and one of the simplest ways to begin a supplement program. Digestive enzymes are necessary for the same reasons. They are no longer in many of our foods, and we can't or don't manufacture, in our bodies, many that we need for proper digestion. But even making good supplement choices can be difficult and often confusing.

It seems like today we are bombarded with supplement choices and claims, but how do we discern which claims we should believe and which supplements would be the best choice for our money? It is important to understand that all supplements are not created equal, and what you get from a discount store, online or from a multi-level company may not be the same as what you might get from a reputable health food store. That being said, it is not as easy as to think that purchasing the most expensive supplement will assure you the best quality supplement. The following are a couple of points to remember that will assist you in choosing the supplements that you can have confidence in their ability to produce the results you are looking for, and in the most cost effect means possible. Many companies, even established health food brands, cannot truthfully claim they regularly use the world's leading ingredients. These brands do not deliver clinically proven European extracts throughout their herbal product line. Additionally, many formulas that appear to contain good ingredients, do not contain the therapeutic levels required to produce results. Many products also fail to verify the potency of a supplement through independent laboratory testing.

The following are a few tips to help assure you get the most out of your vitamin selection and to assist you in choosing quality supplements.

1. Always buy well-known, reputable brands – this is more easily assured when you buy from reputable source like nutrition stores with a knowledgeable staff, willing to assist you in making the best choice for you.

2. Always choose whole food concentrate vitamins, rather than chemical based vitamins.
Food based vitamins are more bioavailable, contain nutrients as they occur in food and are not made from by- products of the petrochemical (or gasoline) refining process.

3. Choose a multi-vitamin that is taken in divided doses throughout the day rather than "one a day".
While it may seem a little less convenient to take three pills as opposed to one, it is necessary to replace certain nutrients throughout the day. Many vitamins are out of your system, or completely used up within hours of ingestion. It doesn't really make much sense to have antioxidant protection for the first three hours of your day, and not the next twenty-one. Time released multivitamins also leave you lacking in nutrients, as vitamins and minerals are absorbed through different points in your digestive system, and often the timed release is "releasing" past its point of absorption.

4. Avoid multivitamins that only offer 100% of the RDA.
The recommended dietary allowances (RDAs) were established more than fifty years ago as the minimum amount of nutrients needed to prevent deficiency diseases in most healthy people. These amounts do not take into account environmental changes and our constant bombardment with pollutants, or individual needs based on age, stress or dietary considerations.

A good example of this would be with Vitamin C. The estimated daily intake of Vitamin C required to prevent Scurvy is between 30-50mg. That is approximately the amount found in one orange, lime or lemon. Years ago, before much was known about the many other biochemical roles of Vitamin C, the RDA for ascorbic acid was set at 60mg, the amount determined to prevent Scurvy. Despite recommendations by the Food & Nutrition Board of the National Academy of Sciences, and the fact that over several decades many scientific studies have shown that optimum health requires many times more than 60mg of Vitamin C, the official RDA remains at 60mg. Considering just one cigarette destroys approximately 500mg. of Vitamin C (this includes second hand smoke), 60mg is well below the minimum necessary for those focusing on optimizing their health.

5. Choose Products Formulated Using the Latest Scientific Evidence

Look for products whose formulators feature some of the most advanced nutrients and botanical ingredients available. I believe it takes three key things to make a nutritional supplement work - Efficacy, Synergy and Bioavailability. There are a few manufactures who have product development teams dedicated to finding the latest discoveries in the supplement world through clinical studies published in scientific journals. Using this information, each ingredient in the formula is included at levels that are proven effective; this is what is known as efficacy. You will also find that these formulas not only feature carefully chosen ingredients, in efficacious amounts, but the most beneficial ingredients combined together work synergistically to enhance the overall effectiveness of the product to produce unrivaled benefits.

6. Look for quality ingredients

Look for products that utilize trademarked or patented ingredients. These ingredients are usually the very ones used in medical research. The companies who manufacture these ingredients conduct scientific research to help establish the safety and efficacy of their ingredients. They also usually use strict quality control procedures to ensure ingredients are free of unwanted impurities and contaminants. Additionally, it is very difficult to achieve consistent quality in the production of herbs and botanical products because of natural variations from plant to plant. Predictable therapeutic results require a strong commitment to expensive and very sophisticated scientific methods and technology. For this rea son, I am particularly partial to European standardized extracts. Europe an governments regulate the quality, safety and effectiveness of herbal products using the same strict standards as used for certain U.S. medica tions. In fact, they categorize botanical extracts as "herbal drugs." There fore, European pharmaceutical companies have a strong commitment to excellence in the botanical sciences, and excel at producing herbal prod ucts of highly consistent quality. Each product is carefully extracted to achieve the optimum levels of biologically active compounds. They are also clinically tested to prove their safety and effectiveness before they are introduced to the marketplace.

But remember, supplements are just that – supplements. They should be taken in addition to, not in place of, an intelligent diet. Supplements will not make up for a diet high in refined carbohydrates, sugars and saturated fats, low in fiber, or a sedentary lifestyle.

As for the discouraging news about our produce, a visit to your local farmers' market is well worth the trip. This is one of the best ways to get vine ripened, fresh picked produce, that is more colorful, flavorful and certainly more nutritious.

Recommended Supplements

*The following products and brands adhere to the quality guidelines as discussed.
These are recommened basic supplements. More specific supplement information can
be found at www.catherinewilbert.com/supplements*

OptiPRO M®️ Functional Shake Protein Mix by PhytoCeutical Formulations

OptiCLA®️ by PhytoCeutical Formulations

Life Essentials Multi-vitamin by Wellness Innovations or similar

Cod Liver Oil, Omega-3, or Complete Omega by Wellness Innovations
    or Nordic Naturals

Coenzyme B-50 Complex by Wellness Innovations or similar

Fiber Fusion (powder) by Enzymatic Therapy or
    Psyllium Husk (powder) by Wellness Innovations or
    Fiber Clean Caps by Wellness Innovations

Ultra Greens by Wellness Innovations or similar
    Earth's Promise Greens by Enzymatic Therapy or

n-Zymax Digestive Enzymes by PhytoCeutical Formulations

Alpha Lipoic Acid by Wellness Innovations or similar

Beta Carotene w/ mixed carotenoids by Wellness Innovations or similar

Supremadopholis probiotic complex by Wellness Innovations or similar

BioActive Glutamine by PhytoCeutical Formulations

Pure Way C 1000 with bioflavanoids by Wellness Innovations or similar

Calcium Magnesium by Wellness Innovations or similar

BioCoQ10 100-200mg by PhytoCeutical Formulations

Kefir - organic and unsweetened by Lifeway

Acai Powder by Sambazon or Navitas

> NOTE: If your favorite health food store doesn't carry these brands,
> ask your trusted wellness consultant to contact these companies or
> recommend their favorite comparable alternative.

THE PLAN

Next few pages are some guidelines and sample meal plans.

If you *really* follow these few sample guidelines you will see results.

These guidelines are proven to work, the only variable in the prelimary results is you! Follow them to success.

Use times on pages to track your meal times.

General Guidelines

- **Eat every 3-4 hours, 5 times per day divided into 3 meals and 2 snacks – all protein based.**

- Always eat a protein rich, well balanced carb/fat meal upon waking and following training. These are your most important meals of the day.

- Always wait at least three hours but never more than four hours between protein based meals.

- Never eat more than one serving (up to 50 grams of protein for men and 35 – 40 grams for women) in one meal.

- Eat only the allocated amounts of each protein: carbohydrates (both complex and simple) and fats.

- **Do not eat complex carbs or sugar at night -- Carbs should come from fibrous carbs -veggies, salads or greens.**

- Fats can be eaten throughout the day – up to 3 servings. Remember, whole eggs, salmon and fatty fish, as well as red meat, all count as 1 serving of fat.

Guidelines for Caloric Breakdown

Breakfast -   Men – 40g protein, 25g of carbs, 10g of fat*
               Women – 25-30g protein, 15-25g carbs, 10g fat*

Snack -   Men – 20-30g protein, 10g of carbs
               Women –10-15g protein, 10g carbs

Lunch -   Men – 40g of protein, 25g carbs, 10g Fat*
               Women – 25-30g protein, 15-25g of carbs, 10g Fat*

Snack -   Men – 20g protein, 10-15g carbs
               Women –10-15g protein, 10g carbs

Dinner -   Men – 40g of protein, 10-15g carbs, 10g Fat*
               Women – 25-30g of protein, 10g carbs, 10g Fat*

*** Fats may be eaten with meals or snacks –
remember to not exceed** recommended daily servings
or your personal recommended daily allotment.
(3 per day - unsaturated, not including supplements,
fish oil and CLA)

SAMPLE MENU GROUPS (WOMEN)

This is just a sampling of menu ideas. For additional menu ideas, log on to
www.catherinewilbert.com/samplemenus

GROUP ONE: Breakfast

(If used for dinner, cut Complex Carb portion.)

Time: _____   **Choose: 1 per day**

1)   1 scoop OptiPRO® protein shake mix with 7-8 oz water (add 1 scoop OptiCLA®)

      *try using 5-6 oz water with 2-3 oz unsweetened Kefir for a creamy "yogurt" shake

      1 slice 7 grain bread or low carb bread

      1 TBL fresh nut butter or Earth Balance® Buttery Spread

2)   6-8 oz non-fat or low carb yogurt

      *try Greek yogurt for a thick "mousse" treat

      ½ - ⅔ scoop OptiPRO® protein shake mix

      ⅛ cup slivered almonds or ¼ cup granola or Zone Cereal

3)   Dr. C's Super Shake Recipe

      There are more nutrients in this shake than most people eat in a day, perhaps a week. What a way to start your day !

      8 oz. Water*
      3 oz. Lifeway plain, unsweetened organic Kefir
      1 scoop OptiPro M Strawberry protein shake – mix
      1 heaping teaspoon Acai Powder or mixed Super Food Powder
      1 heaping teaspoon Maca Powder
      1 heaping teaspoon Ultra Greens Powder
      1 heaping teaspoon sprouted, or milled flax meal
      1 scoop OptiCLA Powder
      2-3 ice cubes to chill
      Shake and enjoy

      For ease and speed, this shake is easily made in a shaker cup – if your choose, you may prepare it in a blender and add a cup of ice.

      Water may be adjusted up or down for desired thickness of shake.

GROUP ONE: Breakfast   *continued*

---

4)   ½ cup oatmeal or 1 packet Natures Path Instant Oatmeal

½ - ⅔ scoop of Vanilla OptiPRO® protein shake mix added to cereal or as a shake

(see item 1)

5)   Soy protein shake made with the following:

1 heaping scoop of OptiPRO® protein shake mix

6 – 8 oz Silk soy milk (or 4 oz water & 4 oz plain organic Kefir)

1 cup frozen organic blueberries and/or strawberries

6)   Omelets made with the following:

6 egg whites or 1 whole egg with 4 whites or 5 egg whites with 1 slice soy cheese, sliced free range turkey/chicken, veggies and salsa

1 slice multi-grain bread

1 TBL Earth Balance® spread

7)   Scrambled eggs with "sausage"

1 whole and 2 whites (May add 2 oz or 1 slice soy or rice cheese.)

2 Boca breakfast patties or Gimme Lean sausage

Try wrapping it in a Fat Flush Tortilla & add salsa..."mmm."*

8)   ⅔ cup Zone Cereal or Kays naturals protein cereal & ⅓ – ½ cup any Peace or Nature's Path® Cereals or granola with 4 – 6 oz Silk soy milk or 2 oz Kefir & 3 oz soy milk

9)   1 cup nonfat cottage cheese with ½ cup nonfat fruit yogurt - may top with low carb granola, nuts or berries.

— — — — *Quick Tip* — — — —

In a hurry? If you are tempted to skip breakfast and run out of the door with just your morning coffee, add a scoop of OptiPRO M® Rich Cocoa or Creamy Vanilla. Now you will have a great tasting breakfast that jump starts your metabolism, stabilizes your blood sugar, and sets you up for better energy for the day!
*Hot coffee is not hot enough to break down protein.

GROUP TWO: Lunch

Feel free to switch out suggested vegetables for seasonal veggies and veggies of your choice. Just be sure to include a green vegetable. Also, season and dress your meals to suit your taste. But stay away from heavy condiments like butter, mayonnaise and creamy or rich dressings.

Try these healthy options:

Butter - Substitute Earth Balance® or non-hydrogenated butter spread

Mayo - Nayonaisse (plain or Dijon style)

Dressing - Bragg Liquid Aminos, Apple Cider Vinegar or organic vinegarette dressing

Time: _____   **Choose: 1 per day**

1) 6 oz grilled free range chicken breast or wild caught fish

6 oz sweet potato

1 cup steamed vegetables (broccoli, cauliflower, green beans, asparagus, spinach)

2) 6 oz grilled wild caught salmon

½ cup brown rice

2 cups steamed vegetables (broccoli, cauliflower, green beans, asparagus, spinach)

3) 6 oz wild caught tuna steak or lean beef (once per week)

6 oz sweet potato

1 cup steamed vegetables (broccoli, cauliflower, green beans, asparagus, spinach)

4) Large Salad with 6 oz grilled chicken or tuna

balsamic vinaigrette dressing on side

GROUP TWO: Lunch   *continued*

---

5)   Stir Fry

6 oz grilled free range chicken breast

½ cup brown rice

2 cups steamed vegetables (broccoli, cauliflower, green beans, asparagus, spinach)

1 TBL olive oil

1 clove garlic

1 TBL soy sauce – low sodium

6)   6 oz free range chicken breast

½ cup brown rice or soy pasta

½ cup fat-free pasta sauce

1 cup steamed vegetables (broccoli, cauliflower, green beans, asparagus, spinach)

7)   1 can Tongal tuna in water with 1-2 TBL Dijon Nayonaise

24 soy crisps or 2 cups of shredded (coleslaw) cabbage

8)   Veggie Burger (Boca) or free range turkey burger on a Rudy's Right Choice bun or an Alvarado Street Bakery sprouted wheat bun with Dijon Nayonaise & low sugar BBQ sauce - add a slice of soy cheese (pepperjack soy is awesome) for a low fat zip with added protein.

GROUP TWO: Lunch *continued*

9) Turkey Wrap with 6 oz free range turkey breast (can substitute turkey for free range chicken, tuna or salmon salad), soy cheese, Dijon Nayonaise, tomatoes, onions, greens, sprouts, ½ TBL sunflower seeds on a low carb wrap. Add 2 oz hummus and baby carrots on the side.

> Note: Look for wrap in which the majority of carbs come from fiber, that are low in sugar, high in protein. "Flat Out-Carb Down" wraps are good choices.

Wraps are so versatile. Feel free to change it up. I like to do a Mediterranean twist by wrapping up free range turkey, hummus, red onion, feta and greens. You could also add olives if you like. Similarly, you can do a southwest take with your wraps by using guacamole, salsa and grated soy cheddar. The trick is to keep it fun and interesting!

---

* Note regarding Complex Carbs and Veggies: Fibrous carbs slow the conversion of complex carbs thus lowering the glycemic index. Therefore, it is a good idea to eat vegetables along with complex carbs – Ex. 1 cup broccoli with 6 oz sweet potato or mixed vegetables with brown rice.

GROUP THREE: Dinner

Feel free to switch out suggested vegetables for seasonal veggies and veggies of your choice. Just be sure to include a green vegetable. Also, season and dress your meals to suit your taste. But stay away from heavy condiments like butter, mayonnaise and creamy or rich dressings.

Time: _____   **Choose: 1 per day**

1)   6 oz grilled free range chicken breast or wild caught fish
2 cups steamed vegetables (broccoli, cauliflower, green beans, asparagus, spinach)
Salad with balsamic vinaigrette (balsamic vinegar and olive oil)

2)   6 oz grilled wild caught salmon
2 cups steamed vegetables (broccoli, cauliflower, green beans, asparagus, spinach)
Salad with balsamic vinaigrette

3)   Large salad
6 oz free range chicken breast or turkey breast, or 1 can Tongal tuna or 6 oz grilled fish on large bed of mixed greens (with onions, mushrooms, peppers if desired)
2 oz pecans or walnuts
2 TBL balsamic vinaigrette dressing

4)   2 veggie burger patties (Yves or Boca – soy protein)
2 cups steamed vegetables (broccoli, cauliflower, green beans, asparagus, spinach)
Salad with balsamic vinaigrette

5)   ½ can of turkey chili with 1-2 veggie dogs and grated soy cheddar

6)   Grilled Fish Tacos (grill 6-8 oz wild caught tilapia or mahi mahi seasoned with lime juice, chili powder, cayenne, and chipotle) with organic salsa, guacamole, grated soy cheddar and lettuce on a whole wheat tortilla.

GROUP FOUR: Snacks

Time:_____, _____, _____

Choose: 2-3 per day from any of the groups below

PROTEIN SHAKES:
- OptiPRO® Shake
- Labrada Lean Body RTD Shakes (½ shake - 20g)
- Muscle Milk RTD Shakes (½ shake or small pkg- 15-20g)
- Syntna 6 Shake
- IsoPure RTD Shakes (½ shake - 20g)

OTHER PROTEIN SNACKS:
- Think Thin Bars
- Cliff Protein Bars
- Stallone's Protein puddings
- Ostrim or turkey jerky
- Kays Natural Protein Snack Chips or cereal
- Non fat greek yogurt

COMBOS *(protein based):* Fats & Carbs may be added to shake
- OptiPRO® Shake or half RTD Shake with 1 serving of nuts (see fats list) or half of one of the bars listed below..
  - Natural Peanut or Almond Bars
  - Organic Food Bars
  - Organic Fiber Bars
- 4 oz hummus with organic baby carrots
- 4 oz free range chicken or tuna salad with Lite Rounds, Wheatines or Glenny's Organic Soy Crisps
- Nut Thins or Soy Crips with 1 TBL organic peanut or almond butter

— — — — *Quick Tip* — — — —

Instead of that blended frozen coffee drink for an 800 calorie mid afternoon snack, try a plain iced coffee with a scoop of OptiPRO M® Creamy Vanilla or Rich Cocoa for a delicious 100 calorie latte that will keep your metabolism burning, your blood sugar stabilized, and help you not eat everything in sight before you eat dinner!

GROUP FIVE: Fats

Choose: 3-4 per day

• NUTS:

⅛ cup (2 TBL) roasted/raw/unsalted of the following:

Peanuts (approx. 10–12 nuts)	Almonds (approx. 8–10 nuts)
Cashews (approx. 12 nuts)	Walnuts (approx. 5–6 nuts)
Pecans (approx. 8 nuts)	Brazil Nuts (approx. 3–4 nuts)

Soynuts (⅓ cup) – also good source of protein

Pumpkin Seeds (2 oz)

• Nut Butter – 1 TBL Unsalted Peanut, Almond or Soy

• Avocado – Half

• Olives - 10

• Olive Oil – 1 TBL

• Coconut Oil - 1 TBL

• OptiCLA® - 4.6 grams (1-7g scoop)

• Ground Flax meal - 1 TBL - sprinkle on salad, cereal or add to shake (good source of Omega 3 Fatty Acids, Fiber & Lignans)

• Fish Oil - Best source of Omega 3's - at least 1 tsp daily

• Wild Caught Fish, good sources of Omega 3 Fatty Acids:

Tuna (6 oz)	Sardines
Salmon (6 oz)	Mackerel
Anchovies	

(*Fats from Fish or red meats counts as 1 serving of fat for one day. In addition to a serving of protein))

SAMPLE MENU GROUPS (MEN)

This is just a sampling of menu ideas. For additional menu ideas, log on to
www.catherinewilbert.com/samplemenus

GROUP ONE: Breakfast

(If used for dinner, cut Complex Carb portion.)

Time: _____   **Choose: 1 per day**

1)   1½ scoop OptiPRO® protein shake mix with 7-8 oz water (add 1 scoop OptiCLA®)

 *Try using 5-6 oz water with 2-3 oz unsweetened Kefir for a creamy "yogurt" shake.

 1 slice 7 grain bread or low carb bread

 1 TBL fresh nut butter or Earth Balance® Buttery Spread

2)   8 oz non-fat or low carb yogurt

 *try Greek yogurt for a thick "mousse" treat

 ¾ -1 scoop OptiPRO® protein shake mix

 ⅛ cup slivered almonds or ¼ cup granola or Zone Cereal

3)   Dr. C's Super Shake Recipe

 There are more nutrients in this shake than most people eat in a day, perhaps a week. What a way to start your day !

 8 oz. Water*
 3 oz. Lifeway plain, unsweetened organic Kefir
 1 scoop OptiPro M Strawberry protein shake – mix
 1 heaping teaspoon Acai Powder or mixed Super Food Powder
 1 heaping teaspoon Maca Powder
 1 heaping teaspoon Ultra Greens Powder
 1 heaping teaspoon sprouted, or milled flax meal
 1 scoop OptiCLA Powder
 2-3 ice cubes to chill
 Shake and enjoy

 For ease and speed, this shake is easily made in a shaker cup – if your choose, you may prepare it in a blender and add a cup of ice.

 Water may be adjusted up or down for desired thickness of shake.

GROUP ONE: Breakfast   *continued*

---

4)   ½ cup oatmeal or 1 packet Natures Path Instant Oatmeal

¾ scoop of Vanilla OptiPRO® protein shake mix added to cereal or as a shake

(see item 1)

5)   Soy protein shake made with the following:

1-2 heaping scoops of OptiPRO® protein shake mix

6 – 8 oz Silk soy milk (or 4 oz water & 4 oz plain organic Kefir)

1 cup frozen organic blueberries and/or strawberries

6)   Omelets made with the following:

8 egg whites or 1 whole egg with 7 whites or 6 egg whites with 1 slice soy cheese, sliced free range turkey/chicken, veggies and salsa

1 slice multi-grain bread

1 TBL Earth Balance® spread

7)   Scrambled eggs with "sausage"

1 whole and 4 whites (May add 2 oz or 1 slice soy or rice cheese.)

2 Boca breakfast patties or Gimme Lean sausage

Try wrapping it in a Fat Flush Tortilla & add salsa..."mmm."*

8)   ⅔ cup Zone Cereal or Kays naturals protein cereal & ⅓ – ½ cup any Peace or Nature's Path® Cereals or granola with 4 – 6 oz Silk soy milk or 2 oz Kefir & 3 oz soy milk

9)   1 cup nonfat cottage cheese with ½ cup nonfat fruit yogurt - may top with low carb granola, nuts, or berries

— — — — *Quick Tip* — — — —

*In a hurry? If you are tempted to skip breakfast and run out of the door with just your morning coffee, add a scoop of OptiPRO M® Rich Cocoa. Now you will have a great tasting breakfast that jump starts your metabolism, stabilizes your blood sugar, and sets you up for better energy for the day! *Hot coffee is not hot enough to break down protein.*

GROUP TWO: Lunch

Feel free to switch out suggested vegetables for seasonal veggies and veggies of your choice. Just be sure to include a green vegetable. Also, season and dress your meals to suit your taste. But stay away from heavy condiments like butter, mayonnaise and creamy or rich dressings.

Try these healthy options:

> Butter - Substitute Earth Balance® or non-hydrogenated butter spread
>
> Mayo - Nayonaisse (plain or Dijon style)
>
> Dressing - Bragg Liquid Aminos, Apple Cider Vinegar or organic vinegarette dressing

Time: _____   **Choose: 1 per day**

1) 8 oz grilled free range chicken breast or wild caught fish

  6 oz sweet potato

  1 cup steamed vegetables (broccoli, cauliflower, green beans, asparagus, spinach)

2) 8 oz grilled wild caught salmon

  ½ cup brown rice

  2 cups steamed vegetables (broccoli, cauliflower, green beans, asparagus, spinach)

3) 8 oz wild caught tuna steak or lean beef (once per week)

  6 oz sweet potato

  1 cup steamed vegetables (broccoli, cauliflower, green beans, asparagus, spinach)

4) Large Salad with 8 oz grilled chicken or tuna

  balsamic vinaigrette dressing on side

GROUP TWO: Lunch   *continued*

___

5)   Stir Fry

        8 oz grilled free range chicken breast

        ½ cup brown rice

        2 cups steamed vegetables (broccoli, cauliflower, green beans,
            asparagus, spinach)

        1 TBL olive oil

        1 clove garlic

        1 TBL soy sauce – low sodium

6)   8 oz free range chicken breast

        ½ cup brown rice or soy pasta

        ½ cup fat-free pasta sauce

        1 cup steamed vegetables (broccoli, cauliflower, green beans,
            asparagus, spinach)

7)   1 can Tongal tuna in water with 1-2 TBL Dijon Nayonaise

        24 soy crisps or 2 cups of shredded (coleslaw) cabbage

8)   Veggie Burger (Boca) or free range turkey burger on a Rudy's Right
        Choice bun or an Alvarado Street Bakery sprouted wheat bun with
        Dijon Nayonaise & low sugar BBQ sauce - add a slice of soy cheese
        (pepperjack soy is awesome) for a low fat zip with added protein.

GROUP TWO: Lunch   *continued*

---

9)   Turkey Wrap with 8 oz free range turkey breast (can substitute turkey
for free range chicken, tuna or salmon salad), soy cheese, Dijon
Nayonaise, tomatoes, onions, greens, sprouts, ½ TBL sunflower
seeds on a low carb wrap. Add 2 oz hummus and baby carrots on the
side.

> Note: Look for wrap in which the majority of carbs
> come from fiber, are low in sugar and high in protein.
> "Flat Out-Carb Down" wraps are good choices.

Wraps are so versatile. Feel free to change it up. I like to do a
Mediterranean twist by wrapping up free range turkey, hummus,
red onion, feta and greens. You could also add olives if you like.
Similarly, you can do a southwest take with your wraps by using
guacamole, salsa and grated soy cheddar. The trick is to keep it fun
and interesting!

---

* Note regarding Complex Carbs and Veggies: Fibrous carbs slow the conversion of
complex carbs thus lowering the glycemic index. Therefore, it is a good idea to eat
vegetables along with complex carbs – Ex. 1 cup broccoli with 6 oz sweet potato or
mixed vegetables with brown rice.

GROUP THREE: Dinner

Feel free to switch out suggested vegetables for seasonal veggies and veggies of your choice. Just be sure to include a green vegetable. Also, season and dress your meals to suit your taste. But stay away from heavy condiments like butter, mayonnaise and creamy or rich dressings.

Time: _____   **Choose: 1 per day**

1) 8 oz grilled free range chicken breast or wild caught fish
   2 cups steamed vegetables (broccoli, cauliflower, green beans, asparagus, spinach)
   Salad with balsamic vinaigrette (balsamic vinegar and olive oil)

2) 8 oz grilled wild caught salmon
   2 cups steamed vegetables (broccoli, cauliflower, green beans, asparagus, spinach)
   Salad with balsamic vinaigrette

3) Large salad
   8 oz free range chicken breast or turkey breast, or 1 can Tongal tuna or 6 oz grilled fish on large bed of mixed greens (with onions, mushrooms, peppers if desired)
   2 oz pecans or walnuts
   2 TBL balsamic vinaigrette dressing

4) 2 veggie burger patties (Yves or Boca – soy protein)
   2 cups steamed vegetables (broccoli, cauliflower, green beans, asparagus, spinach)
   Salad with balsamic vinaigrette

5) ½ can of turkey chili with 1-2 veggie dogs and grated soy cheddar

6) Grilled Fish Tacos (grill 8-10 oz wild caught tilapia or mahi mahi seasoned with lime juice, chili powder, cayenne, and chipotle) with organic salsa, guacamole, grated soy cheddar and lettuce on a whole wheat tortilla.

GROUP FOUR: Snacks

Time:_____, _____, _____

Choose: 2-3 per day from any of the groups below

PROTEIN SHAKES:
- OptiPRO® Shake
- Labrada Lean Body RTD Shakes (½ shake - 20g)
- Muscle Milk RTD Shakes (½ shake or small pkg- 15-20g)
- Syntna 6 Shake
- IsoPure RTD Shakes (½ shake - 20g)

OTHER PROTEIN SNACKS:
- Think Thin Bars
- Cliff Protein Bars
- Stallone's Protein puddings
- Ostrim or turkey jerky
- Kays Naturals protein snack chips or cereals
- Non fat greek yogurt

COMBOS *(protein based):* Fats & Carbs may be added to shake
- OptiPRO® Shake or half RTD Shake with 1 serving of nuts (see fats list) or half of one of the bars listed below..
    - Natural Peanut or Almond Bars
    - Organic Food Bars
    - Organic Fiber Bars
- 4 oz hummus with organic baby carrots
- 4 oz free range chicken or tuna salad with Lite Rounds, Wheatines or Glenny's Organic Soy Crisps
- Nut Thins or soy crisps with 1 TBL organic peanut or almond butter

— — — — *Quick Tip* — — — —

Instead of that blended frozen coffee drink for an 800 calorie mid afternoon snack, try a plain iced coffee with a scoop of OptiPRO M® Creamy Vanilla or Rich Cocoa for a delicious 100 calorie latte that will keep your metabolism burning, your blood sugar stabilized, and help you not eat everything in sight before you eat dinner!

GROUP FIVE: Fats

Choose: 3-4per day

• NUTS:

⅛ cup (2 TBL) roasted/raw/unsalted of the following:

    Peanuts (approx. 10–12 nuts)   Almonds (approx. 8–10 nuts)

    Cashews (approx. 12 nuts)   Walnuts (approx. 5–6 nuts)

    Pecans (approx. 8 nuts)   Brazil Nuts (approx. 3–4 nuts)

    Soynuts (⅓ cup) – also good source of protein

    Pumpkin Seeds (2 oz)

• Nut Butter – 1 TBL Unsalted Peanut, Almond or Soy

• Avocado – Half

• Olives - 10

• Olive Oil – 1 TBL

• Coconut Oil - 1 TBL

• OptiCLA® - 4.6 grams (1-7g scoop)

• Ground Flax meal - 1 TBL - sprinkle on salad, cereal or add to shake

    (good source of Omega 3 Fatty Acids, Fiber & Lignans)

• Fish Oil - Best source of Omega 3's - at least 1 tsp daily

• Wild Caught Fish, good sources of Omega 3 Fatty Acids:

    Tuna (6 oz)   Sardines

    Salmon (6 oz)   Mackerel

    Anchovies

    (*Fats from Fish or red meats counts as 1 serving of fat for one day.

        In addition to a serving of protein)

MENDING YOUR METABOLISM

Personal Progress
Journal

Additional journal pages may be downloaded at
www.catherinewilbert.com/journal

Date _____

Time	Food	Calories	Protein	Carbs	Fat	Supplements
Totals						

Activity:

Weight Training

Cardio

Water Consumption:

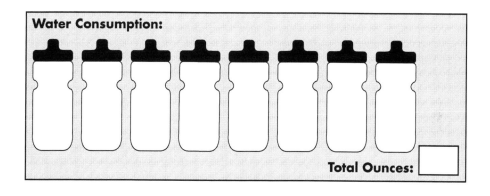

Total Ounces:

Notes:

Date _____

Time	Food	Calories	Protein	Carbs	Fat	Supplements
Totals						

Activity:

Weight Training

Cardio

Water Consumption:

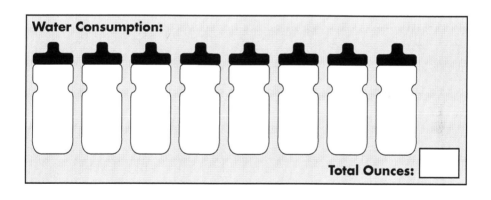

Total Ounces:

Notes:

Date _____

MENDING YOUR METABOLISM

Time	Food	Calories	Protein	Carbs	Fat	Supplements
Totals						

Activity:

Weight Training

Cardio

Water Consumption:

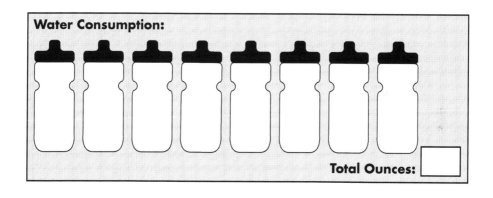

Total Ounces:

Notes:

Date _____

Time	Food	Calories	Protein	Carbs	Fat	Supplements
Totals						

Activity:

Weight Training

Cardio

Water Consumption:

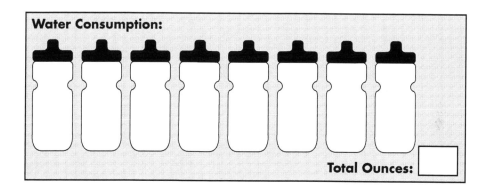

Total Ounces:

Notes:

Date _____

Time	Food	Calories	Protein	Carbs	Fat	Supplements
Totals						

Activity:

Weight Training

Cardio

Water Consumption:

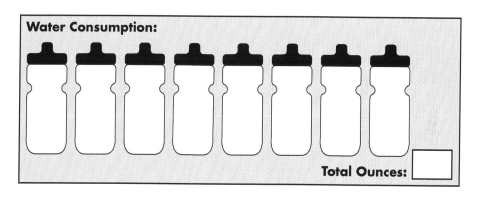

Total Ounces:

Notes:

Date _____

Time	Food	Calories	Protein	Carbs	Fat	Supplements
Totals						

MENDING YOUR METABOLISM

Activity:

Weight Training

Cardio

Water Consumption:

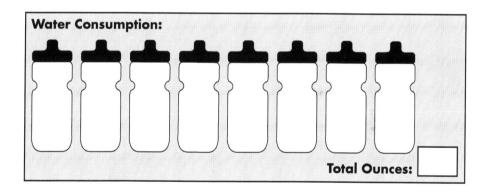

Total Ounces:

Notes:

Date _____

Time	Food	Calories	Protein	Carbs	Fat	Supplements
Totals						

Activity:

Weight Training

Cardio

Water Consumption:

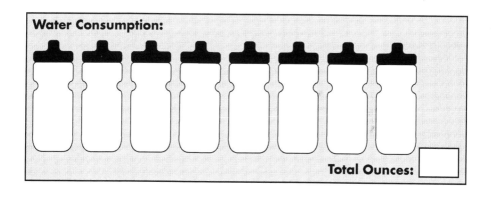

Total Ounces:

Notes:

Date _____

Time	Food	Calories	Protein	Carbs	Fat	Supplements
Totals						

Activity:

Weight Training

Cardio

Water Consumption:

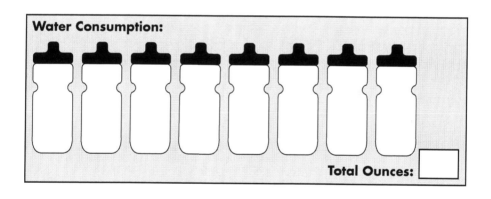

Total Ounces:

Notes:

Date _____

Time	Food	Calories	Protein	Carbs	Fat	Supplements
Totals						

MENDING YOUR METABOLISM

Activity:

Weight Training

Cardio

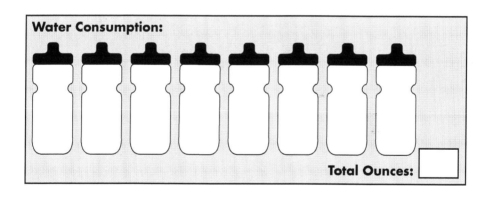

Water Consumption:

Total Ounces:

Notes:

Date _____   MENDING YOUR METABOLISM

Time	Food	Calories	Protein	Carbs	Fat	Supplements
Totals						

Activity:

Weight Training

Cardio

Water Consumption:

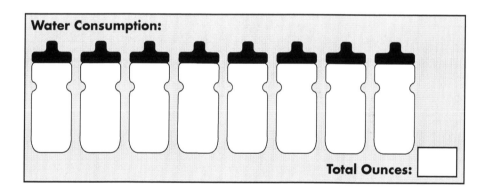

Total Ounces:

Notes:

Date _____

Time	Food	Calories	Protein	Carbs	Fat	Supplements
Totals						

MENDING YOUR METABOLISM

Activity:

Weight Training

Cardio

Water Consumption:

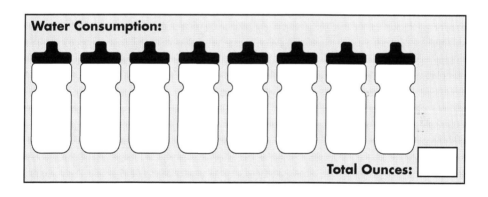

Total Ounces:

Notes:

Date _____

Time	Food	Calories	Protein	Carbs	Fat	Supplements
Totals						

Activity:

Weight Training

Cardio

Water Consumption:

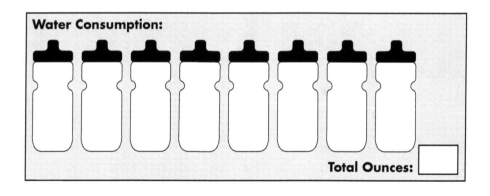

Total Ounces:

Notes:

Date _____

Time	Food	Calories	Protein	Carbs	Fat	Supplements
Totals						

Activity:

Weight Training

Cardio

Water Consumption:

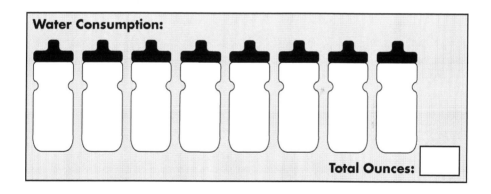

Total Ounces:

Notes:

Time	Food	Calories	Protein	Carbs	Fat	Supplements
Totals						

Activity:

Weight Training

Cardio

Water Consumption:

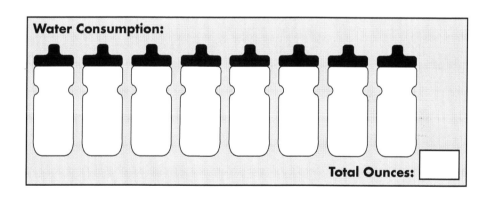

Total Ounces:

Notes:

Date _____

Time	Food	Calories	Protein	Carbs	Fat	Supplements
Totals						

Activity:

Weight Training

Cardio

Water Consumption:

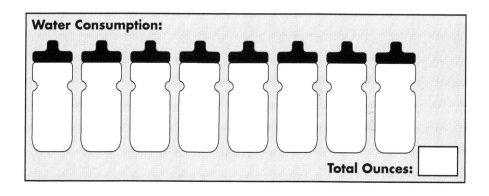

Total Ounces:

Notes:

Date _____

Time	Food	Calories	Protein	Carbs	Fat	Supplements
Totals						

Activity:

Weight Training

Cardio

Water Consumption:

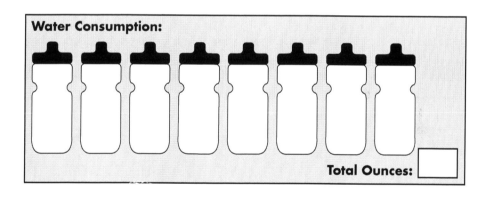

Total Ounces:

Notes:

Date _____

MENDING YOUR METABOLISM

Time	Food	Calories	Protein	Carbs	Fat	Supplements
Totals						

Activity:

Weight Training

Cardio

Water Consumption:

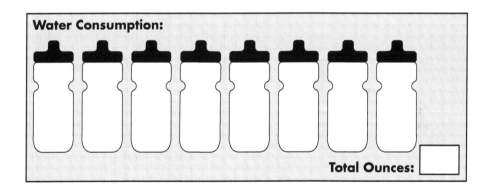

Total Ounces:

Notes:

Date _____

MENDING YOUR METABOLISM

Time	Food	Calories	Protein	Carbs	Fat	Supplements
Totals						

Activity:

Weight Training

Cardio

Water Consumption:

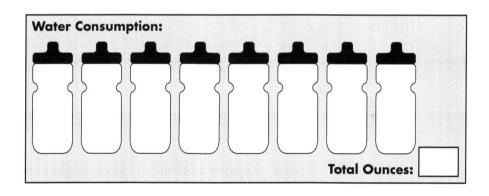

Total Ounces:

Notes:

Date _____

Time	Food	Calories	Protein	Carbs	Fat	Supplements
Totals						

Activity:

Weight Training

Cardio

Water Consumption:

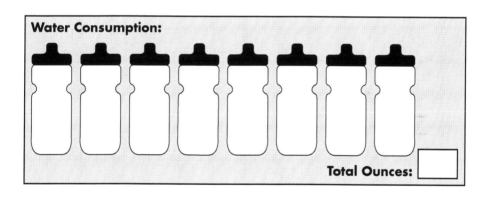

Total Ounces:

Notes:

Date _____

Time	Food	Calories	Protein	Carbs	Fat	Supplements
Totals						

Activity:

Weight Training

Cardio

Water Consumption:

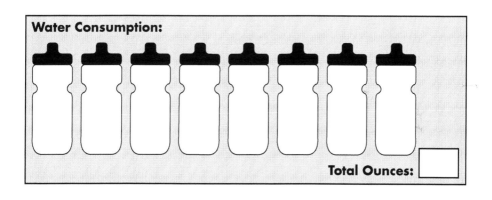

Total Ounces:

Notes:

Date _____

Time	Food	Calories	Protein	Carbs	Fat	Supplements
Totals						

Activity:

Weight Training

Cardio

Water Consumption:

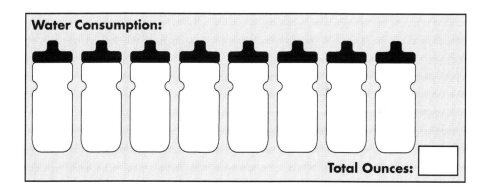

Total Ounces:

Notes:

Time	Food	Calories	Protein	Carbs	Fat	Supplements
Totals						

Activity:

Weight Training

Cardio

Water Consumption:

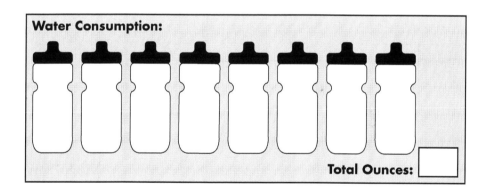

Total Ounces:

Notes:

Date _____

MENDING YOUR METABOLISM

Time	Food	Calories	Protein	Carbs	Fat	Supplements
Totals						

Activity:

Weight Training
Cardio

Water Consumption:

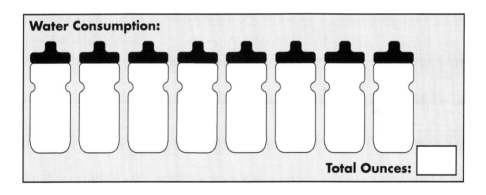

Total Ounces:

Notes:

Date _____

Time	Food	Calories	Protein	Carbs	Fat	Supplements
Totals						

Activity:

Weight Training

Cardio

Water Consumption:

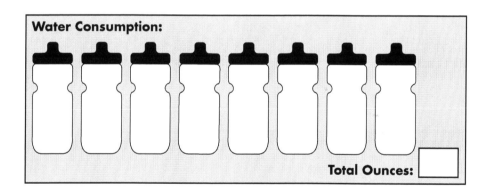

Total Ounces:

Notes:

Date _____

Time	Food	Calories	Protein	Carbs	Fat	Supplements
Totals						

Activity:

Weight Training

Cardio

Water Consumption:

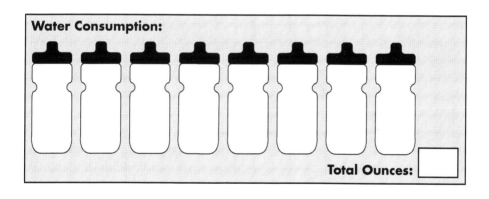

Total Ounces:

Notes:

Date _____

Time	Food	Calories	Protein	Carbs	Fat	Supplements
Totals						

Activity:

Weight Training

Cardio

Water Consumption:

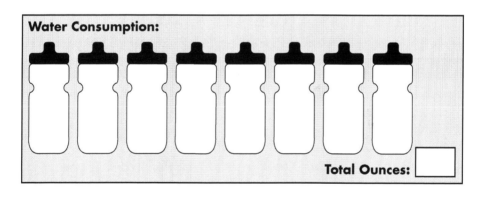

Total Ounces:

Notes:

Date _____

Time	Food	Calories	Protein	Carbs	Fat	Supplements
Totals						

Activity:

Weight Training

Cardio

Water Consumption:

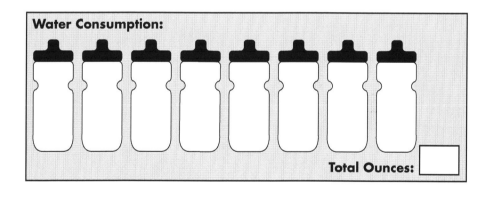

Total Ounces:

Notes:

Date _____

Time	Food	Calories	Protein	Carbs	Fat	Supplements
Totals						

Activity:

Weight Training

Cardio

Water Consumption:

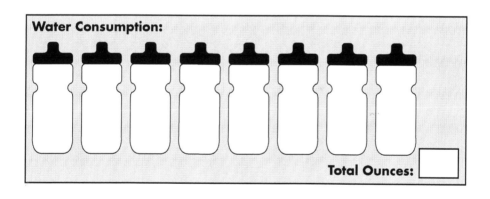

Total Ounces:

Notes:

Date _____

Time	Food	Calories	Protein	Carbs	Fat	Supplements
Totals						

MENDING YOUR METABOLISM

Activity:

Weight Training

Cardio

Water Consumption:

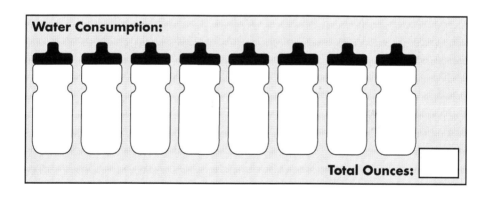

Total Ounces:

Notes:

Date _____

Time	Food	Calories	Protein	Carbs	Fat	Supplements
Totals						

Activity:

Weight Training

Cardio

Water Consumption:

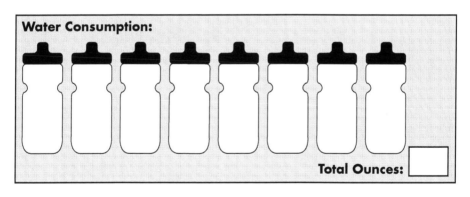

Total Ounces:

Notes:

Date _____

Time	Food	Calories	Protein	Carbs	Fat	Supplements
Totals						

Activity:

Weight Training

Cardio

Water Consumption:

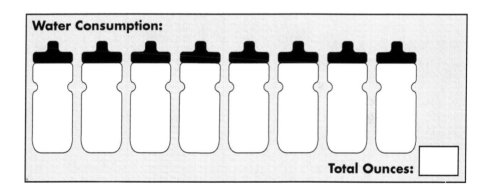

Total Ounces:

Notes:

Date _____

Time	Food	Calories	Protein	Carbs	Fat	Supplements
Totals						

Activity:

Weight Training

Cardio

Water Consumption:

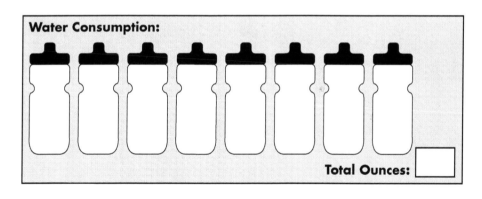

Total Ounces:

Notes:

Date _____

Time	Food	Calories	Protein	Carbs	Fat	Supplements
Totals						

Activity:

Weight Training

Cardio

Water Consumption:

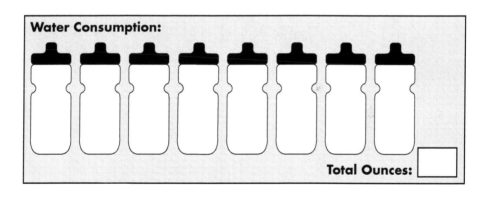

Total Ounces:

Notes:

Date _____

Time	Food	Calories	Protein	Carbs	Fat	Supplements
Totals						

Activity:

Weight Training

Cardio

Water Consumption:

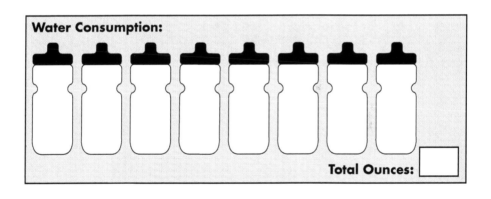

Total Ounces:

Notes:

Date _____

MENDING YOUR METABOLISM

Time	Food	Calories	Protein	Carbs	Fat	Supplements
Totals						

Activity:

Weight Training

Cardio

Water Consumption:

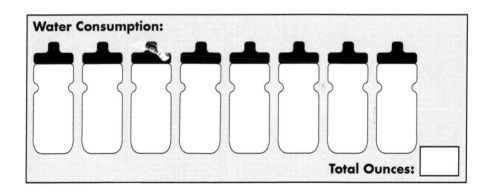

Total Ounces:

Notes:

Date _____

Time	Food	Calories	Protein	Carbs	Fat	Supplements
Totals						

MENDING YOUR METABOLISM

Activity:

Weight Training

Cardio

Water Consumption:

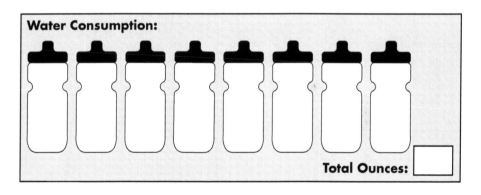

Total Ounces:

Notes:

Date _____

Time	Food	Calories	Protein	Carbs	Fat	Supplements
Totals						

Activity:

Weight Training

Cardio

Water Consumption:

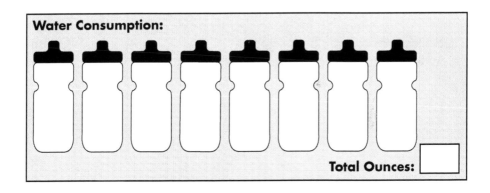

Total Ounces:

Notes:

Date _____

MENDING YOUR METABOLISM

Time	Food	Calories	Protein	Carbs	Fat	Supplements
Totals						

Activity:

Weight Training

Cardio

Water Consumption:

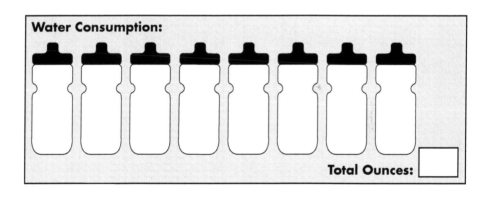

Total Ounces:

Notes:

Date _____   MENDING YOUR METABOLISM

Time	Food	Calories	Protein	Carbs	Fat	Supplements
Totals						

Activity:

Weight Training

Cardio

Water Consumption:

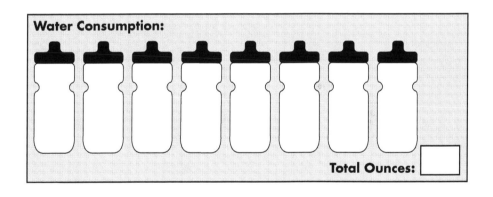

Total Ounces:

Notes:

Date _____

Time	Food	Calories	Protein	Carbs	Fat	Supplements
Totals						

MENDING YOUR METABOLISM

Activity:

Weight Training

Cardio

Water Consumption:

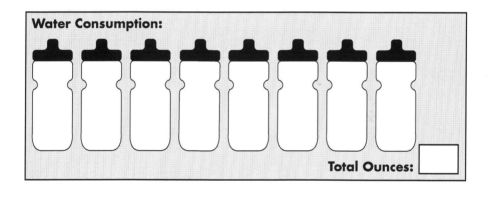

Total Ounces:

Notes:

Date _____

Time	Food	Calories	Protein	Carbs	Fat	Supplements
Totals						

MENDING YOUR METABOLISM

Activity:

Weight Training

Cardio

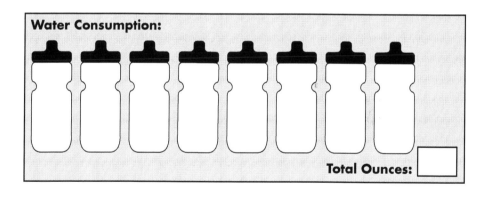

Water Consumption:

Total Ounces:

Notes:

NOTES:

NOTES:

Catherine Wilbert, N.D.

Catherine is a Doctor of Naturopathic Medicine, Nutrition Consultant, Culinary Nutrition Expert & Nationally Recognized Weight Loss & Wellness Expert.

Helping others reach their fitness goals and find new quality of life through health and nutrition has always been a passion for Catherine. This commitment to fitness is not only evident through her dozen bodybuilding titles, which include three national championships, but through her promotion of health and wellness through everything from seminars to national television segments. Through individual consultation, Catherine educates people on the importance of nutrition in the prevention and treatment of illness. She successfully works with people in everything from weight loss to wellness.

She is the owner of The Nutrition Company and Vitality Juice, Java and Smoothie Bar, a growing group of retail nutritional supplement stores offering nutrition, health and wellness education services. Vitality Juice, Java and Smoothie Bar is a groundbreaking concept offering functional foods and beverages, all-natural smoothies, and an organic coffee and juice bar. Her original formulations and recipes have truly broken the old adage that if it is good for you, it doesn't taste good. Catherine prides herself on the fact that there is finally a place where healthy really does taste good. The Vitality Juice Java and Smoothie Bar concept is currently being offered as a franchise opportunity.

As owner, president, and product developer for PhytoCeutical Formulations, Dr. Wilbert has also combined her nutritional and pharmaceutical knowledge with her experience as an athlete to formulate a unique line of nutritional products to provide specific nutritional results and broad ranging, multiple health benefits. PhytoCeutical Formulations products are sold in hundreds of stores across the United States and are in distribution nationally and internationally. Dr. Wilbert is the creator of Swerve™, all natural sugar alternative. Swerve™ is a revolutionary and truly unique sugar alternative that is unlike anything in the marketplace. Swerve™ is an all-natural sweetener that looks, tastes, measures, cooks and bakes just like sugar. It has zero calories, zero glycemic index, and is appropriate for diabetics along with any and everyone wishing to reduce their sugar intake for better weight management and better overall health.

Catherine hosts the weekly talk radio show Natural Wellness, where she answers questions on health, fitness and nutrition and has also served as the wellness expert for several web sites, as well as other weekly radio shows. Dr. Wilbert has appeared as the health and wellness expert on NBC television affiliates across the country and has done a multitude of health related stories for television. She also contributes monthly as nutrition and wellness expert and has been featured in numerous publications.

Dr. Wilbert is available for individual consultations, speaking engagements, seminars, and lectures. She can be reached via email at her website **www.catherinewilbert.com** or by callling **888.551.10180**

3762322